KETO FITNESS

The Ketogenic Diet, Bodybuilding and Strength Training

This book includes:

(1) The Ketogenic Diet: *The Fast Way to Burning Fat*

(2) Bodybuilding: *How to Build the Body of a Greek God*

(3) Strength Training (Secrets): *The Best Tips and Strategies for Getting Stronger*

By Epic Rios

D1508042

Intro

Thanks for purchasing *Keto Fitness: The Ketogenic Diet, Bodybuilding and Strength Training.*

Before you begin reading *Keto Fitness,* make sure you take the time to read over the "Health and Fitness Chief Aim."

The "Health and Fitness Chief Aim" is a unique goal seeking tool designed to help you achieve your health and fitness goals.

Make sure to read over the instructions for the "Health and Fitness Chief Aim" and follow them correctly for creating your very own "Health and Fitness Chief Aim."

In case you forget to read over the "Health and Fitness Chief Aim," it will be provided to you again at the end of this book.

Thanks again for purchasing *Keto Fitness: The Ketogenic Diet, Bodybuilding and Strength Training.*

I wish you great success with achieving your health and fitness goals.

Health and Fitness
Chief Aim

*Use the following guide for achieving your health and fitness goals.

Step #1

Write down your health and fitness goal(s) and be specific. For example, if you want to lose 10 pounds then write down, "I want to lose 10 pounds."

At the same time, if you want to build muscle, be specific and write down the amount of muscle you want to have. For example, if you want to have 10 pounds of muscle then write down, "I want to have 10 pounds of muscle."

Step #2

Write down the date by which you want to achieve your health and fitness goal(s).

For example, "I will lose 10 pounds by February 2019."

Example two, "I will be able to run 15 miles nonstop by May 2019."

Step 3

Write down what you are willing to sacrifice in order to achieve your health and fitness goals. In addition, write down what are you willing to give back (to the world) in return for achieving your health and fitness goal(s).

For example, "I am willing to give up drinking alcohol, specifically beer for the next 3 months in order to lose 20 pounds of fat. In addition, I am going to stop watching television after 10:00 PM and I will instead go to sleep early so that I can wake up early and exercise."

"In return for achieving my health and fitness goals, I will serve as a role model inspiring and helping others to also achieve their health and fitness goals by sharing my knowledge, experience and wisdom."

Step 4

Repeat looking and reading over your Health and Fitness Chief Aim every day until you achieve your health and fitness goals. In addition, look and read over your Health and Fitness Chief Aim multiple times a day. Daily repetition is important for achieving any goal.

THE KETOGENIC DIET

The Fast Way to Burning Fat

By Epic Rios

"Pursue your health and fitness goals diligently, patiently and persistently and you are bound to be successful."   *– Epic Rios*

Table of Contents

Introduction

Congratulations on purchasing this book and thank you for doing so. The following chapters will discuss what you need to know to get started on the ketogenic diet.

This diet plan is one of the best diet plans out there because it is effective and it helps you to lose weight and burn off that stubborn fat that you have been working against for a long time.

Simply this effective book will provide you with all of the information that you need to fully understand and follow the ketogenic diet plan.

We will start out with some of the basics of the ketogenic diet, the benefits of this diet plan, how to eat properly, the best meal plans to help you get started, how the ketogenic diet and intermittent fasting can work together, and even how you can modify this diet plan for your workout plan.

Anyone is able to follow the ketogenic diet, and with the help of this educational book, you will be able to see amazing results with your fat and weight loss in no time.

When you have been trying other diet plans for some time and are not seeing the results that you would like, it may be time to change things up and try something new.

The ketogenic diet will effectively help you to see the results that you would like, and this resourceful book will give you all the information that you need to get started.

I want to take the time to thank you so much for choosing this book! Every effort was made to ensure it is full of as much useful information as possible, please enjoy!

Chapter 1: What is the Ketogenic Diet?

When you are ready to get started on a new diet plan, there are a lot of different options that you can choose from.

Some diets are going to be more like "fasting" where you need to cut out what you eat so much that it is very hard to stick with it.

Other diets will focus on cutting out all of the fats that you consume during the day so that you can focus on eating healthy carbs and lots of fruits and vegetables in your diet.

Some diets are healthy and some are not that healthy and there are often many people who swear by these healthy and unhealthy diets.

But think about this, which diet is actually going to give you the best results that you would like to practice when it comes to losing weight?

It is important to state that the ketogenic diet is one of the most effective diet plans that you can choose from.

The ketogenic diet plan is simple to understand.

In addition, learning and practicing the ketogenic diet is going to take away some of the common misconceptions about dieting, the misconceptions that have been holding you back from losing weight so that you can actually achieve your fat loss goals.

While many traditional diets, the ones that are considered really healthy, will ask you to eat more carbs and cut down on fats, the ketogenic diet takes things in a different direction.

With the ketogenic diet, you are going to severely limit the carbs that you take in and instead replace them with healthy fats that will increase your metabolism and make you feel amazing in no time.

The issue with normal diet plans is that you are taking in too many carbs. These carbs may seem healthy, but when the body breaks them down, they basically become sugars in the body.

If you are consuming additional foods that have sugars in them then this could add some additional issues to your health and prevent you from achieving your weight loss goals.

Keep this in mind - the body is used to consuming carbs for energy. So, the body is very happy when you take in some carbs and the body will use the carbs for energy.

The body will then transfer the carbs over to insulin and then try to use up the insulin. And when the body doesn't use up all of its insulin, then the body simply stores it as fat. As a result, a person will simply gain weight or not be able to lose fat as a result of the excess insulin.

Unfortunately, carbs are a very effective source of energy for most people. The body will often feel hungry and run down long before you use up the carbs that you consume, and you will eventually feel tired, grumpy, and hungry again.

This leads most people to eat more carbs in an effort to get their energy back.

After eating more carbs, people will feel better for a little while. But soon they will be tired and worn out again and the cycle just keeps going on and on.

Eventually you will end up eating way too many calories just to keep your energy levels up and all those extra carbs will be stored as excess body fat.

The ketogenic diet works to break this cycle. Instead of relying so much on eating carbs, you will instead rely on eating healthy fats.

You can still have some carbs, but the point is to push your body into **ketosis, a process where the body will use fats instead of carbs as its main source of energy**.

It is important to state that fat or "healthy fat" can be a really efficient source of energy.

While you will feel worn out and tired for the first few days as the body runs out of carbs (due to you eating fewer carbs), and starts looking for a new energy source, you will soon notice that your energy levels will start to go through the roof.

You will burn the "healthy fat" that you are eating as well as the "fats" that are stored in the body, all while feeling full and satisfied.

When you go on the ketogenic diet, you are responsible for cutting down the number of carbs that you consume.

On the ketogenic diet, most people will be limited to eating no more than fifty grams of carbs each day. In addition, most of these carbs will come from healthy sources like fruits and vegetables.

Some people like to push themselves into ketosis a little bit faster and will limit themselves to twenty grams of carbs a day or less.

However, it is advisable to slowly begin the ketogenic diet and to also slowly begin to reduce the number of carbs you eat each day.

Every person that practices the ketogenic diet needs to experiment with their carb intake based on their activity levels and other factors.

For example, people who do a lot of weightlifting, aerobics and cardio based exercises (swimming, running, etc.,) will need to take in slightly more carbs or above the fifty-gram recommendation to help them stay healthy and so that they can maintain being in ketosis.

(Ketosis is a process by which the body uses stored fat or body fat as fuel or energy. So, when very little carbs are consumed and that energy is used up, the body will go into ketosis in which the body will look to fat as an energy source for using as fuel or energy.)

Checking to see if you are in ketosis is very important if you are practicing the ketogenic diet.

You will only lose weight once you reach the state of ketosis and some people may need to adjust their food intake a bit more than others to see some weight loss results.

It is important to state that there are test strips available at pharmacies that you can buy that will allow you to check for the level of ketones in your body, so that you can adjust your diet early on and figure out what changes you need to make to your diet.

(Ketones are chemical substances that the body produces when there is not enough insulin produced in the body as a result of eating very few carbs.

So, the less carbs you eat the less insulin your body will produce resulting in ketones being produced by the body. So, ketones occur as a result of the body using fat as energy or fuel.)

Remember that when working with the ketogenic diet, you need to change up the way that you are eating on a regular basis.

You are not going to be able to eat a ton of bread and pasta and see results. However, lots of healthy oils and fats from healthy protein sources can help you to get the macronutrients that you need and to lose weight.

Carbs are not completely off limits, but you will be surprised at how quickly your daily allowance will disappear, especially if you are choosing bread and pasta as your carb sources.

Instead, you need to stick with healthy fruits and vegetables and learn how to go with the ones that are lower in carb content compared to others.

This makes it easier to get the vitamins and nutrients that your body needs without pushing the body out of ketosis.

Once you reach ketosis through healthy fats, moderate amounts of protein, and low carbs, you will need to maintain this diet for the long-term. As soon as you start to eat more carbs and go back to your old habits, you will get out of ketosis and can start to gain the weight again.

You can easily lose a lot of weight with the ketogenic diet, but you need to maintain the ketosis diet for the long-term if you really want to see the good results.

Following the ketogenic diet can be a bit difficult for some people. You may have to give up some of the foods that you have enjoyed in the past.

But once you learn a few of the rules that come with the ketogenic diet and you find a few favorite recipes that will help you to stay within the right macronutrient content for your body and for ketosis you are going to fall in love with the results.

The ketogenic diet may be hard in our modern world, but it is going to give you some amazing results with your weight and fat loss goals.

Understanding Ketosis

Ketosis is basically the process of your body relying on fats rather than on carbs or glucose to provide it with energy.

Most people eat enough carbs that they are going to rely on those for their source of energy. But this is not a very efficient form of energy.

You will quickly go through cycles of high energy and then crash when the carbs are all gone, and you will end up eating way more than you need just to keep your energy levels up.

With ketosis, you do not need to worry about your energy levels crashing and then trying to eat more carbs in order to increase your energy levels again.

Instead, you will teach the body to stop relying on carbs and instead the body will learn to rely on healthy fats that you start to take in.

When you eat healthy fats, ketones are going to be produced and used for energy.

Ketones will replace the glucose, giving you plenty of healthy energy without having to worry about the horrible crashes that glucose (sugars from carbs) causes.

Eating on the Ketogenic Diet

When you follow a ketogenic diet, you will consume at least 70 percent of your calories each day from fat.

The majority of the rest will come from protein, with only about five percent coming from healthy sources of carbs, such as low-carb vegetables.

As a beginner, you will need to build your meals around healthy sources of fats. These can include oils, cheese, nuts, meats, and fatty fish.

You can then add in some healthy sources of protein if they are not included already, as well as healthy low-carb options like vegetables and some fruits.

One thing to keep in mind on this diet plan is that you still need to take in moderate amounts of protein.

Many people get so focused on the fat intake and limiting their carbs that they forget to take in enough protein.

Protein is important to help you stay full and for preserving your body's muscles as well as keeping your muscles strong.

Negative Effects of This Diet Plan

You may also wonder if there are any negative effects of following this diet plan. Plain and simple, you are taking a large food group (carbs) and cutting it down to almost nothing on this diet plan.

For the most part, as soon as your body has time to adapt to ketosis, there shouldn't be any negative effects that you need to deal with.

You may feel a bit tired in the beginning as your body adapts, but once that adaption happens, you will find that you have more energy than ever before.

You should make sure that you have a wide variety of food options when it comes to eating on the ketogenic diet plan.

If you eat the same meals each day, or the same vegetables, you are going to miss out on important nutrients and this can cause some negative effects.

This is true of any diet plan if you do not add in variety. Make sure that you get plenty of variety in the diet, and you will see amazing results without any negative side effects.

Do I Need to Measure Ketones?

Many people choose to monitor the ketones that they consume. Actually, it is important that you monitor your ketones in order to ensure that you reach ketosis and that you stay within it to see weight loss results.

It is not necessarily a requirement for the diet plan, but it certainly helps. Measuring your ketones does not have to be difficult.

There are some testing strips that you can use that will tell you when you have entered ketosis and you can bring these out any time that you are worried about whether you are in the right range with your carbs or not.

Who Uses the Ketogenic Diet?

The biggest reason that people will choose to go on the ketogenic diet is to simply lose weight.

When you start relying on fat for your source of energy rather than glucose (sugars), you can melt off the weight and fat in no time.

However, there are many other reasons that people may choose to practice the ketogenic diet.

Originally, the ketogenic diet was designed to help patients who were dealing with a variety of neurological conditions, especially epilepsy.

It was found that young children who relied on a ketogenic-like diet were able to reduce the frequency of their seizures and reduce their medications.

Believe it or not, but there are some athletes who like to use the ketogenic diet to help with their endurance.

According to a paper that was released in the European Journal of Clinical Nutrition, there are a few other reasons that someone may choose to use the ketogenic diet.

These include:

- Evidence that the ketogenic diet can help people with high cholesterol, type 2 diabetes, weight loss, and epilepsy.

- New evidence has shown how the ketogenic diet may be able to help with a variety of neurological diseases like brain trauma, narcolepsy, Alzheimer's, and Parkinson's Disease, to name a few.

- People that suffer from cancer, severe acne, and even polycystic ovarian syndrome are often helped with the ketogenic diet as well.

Basically, anyone is able to use the ketogenic diet, whether they want to lose weight or are working to avoid one of the conditions named above.

The ketogenic diet is easy to follow and gives such amazing benefits to those who are able to follow it.

Chapter 2: The Benefits of the Ketogenic Diet

There are a lot of reasons that people will choose to use and practice the ketogenic diet. Simply, the ketogenic diet is one of the most effective diet plans out there.

In addition, the ketogenic diet can help resolve a variety of health issues that people are dealing with and not just with weight loss.

Some of the great benefits that you will receive when you decide to use and practice the ketogenic diet are:

- **Lose weight:** The number one reason that people choose to use the ketogenic diet is that they want to lose weight. And this diet plan is very effective at helping this to happen.

  Once your body enters into the process of ketosis and starts relying on fats for energy rather than carbs, you will see the weight melt off in no time.

- **Next, the ketogenic diet can help reduce cancer:** Some studies have shown how the ketogenic diet may be effective at reducing your risks of developing cancer.

  Cancer cells thrive when given lots of carbs, so if you take these carbs away, they will basically starve out. Regular healthy cells can rely on healthy fats for their nutrition, but cancer cells can't.

- **Next, the ketogenic diet will give you more energy:** During the first few days on the ketogenic diet, you may notice that you are feeling tired and worn down. This is because the body is so used to relying on carbs to stay energetic.

  When you take those carbs away, the body is not sure where to find its energy source and may feel run down.

  You just need to give it a few days, though; the body will start using the fats that you provide it for energy in no time. Once that happens, you will have more energy than ever before.

- **Next, the ketogenic diet will help lower your risk of diabetes:** With all those carbs you traditionally eat, it is common to see a risk of diabetes.

  You have to be very careful of the carbs you eat because the body will treat some carbs you eat just like sugars once they are eaten and broken down.

  So, if you are eating some sugars and lots of carbs, you are raising your insulin levels and increasing the amount of risk you have for diabetes.

  Cut out a lot of those carbs, as well as the sugars, and your body can clean itself up and cut down on your risk of diabetes.

- **Next, the ketogenic diet will lower your blood pressure:** Many people who have gone on the ketogenic diet report that their blood pressures went down.

  Many of the foods that you consume on a regular diet will have a ton of sodium inside, which can raise your blood pressure.

Add in all the processed foods, high amount of carbs, and even the bad fats, and it is no wonder that most people have bad high blood pressure.

The ketogenic diet cuts out a lot of these bad unhealthy foods out of your diet so that you can recover and get that blood pressure back to normal.

- **Next, the ketogenic diet is great for the heart:** The ketogenic diet can even help out with the health of your heart.

  The healthy fats that you consume will help to strengthen your heart. The healthy fats also deliver some of those healthy vitamins and nutrients over to the heart better than carbs do.

  So, once you are reducing some of the carbs, the ones that turn into sugars in the body, you are giving the heart a fighting chance to be healthy and strong again.

- **Next, the ketogenic diet clears the mind:** When you are able to cut down on the number of carbs that you consume, and the number of calories that you are consuming, you will find that your mind feels much clearer.

  It will feel amazing to remember things, to think things through critically, and to no longer have to deal with the brain fog that you may have suffered from before as a result of eating so many carbs.

- **Next, the ketogenic diet can help fight epilepsy:** Originally, the ketogenic diet was developed as a way to help children who were suffering from chronic epilepsy.

The high fat and low carb ketogenic diet were effective at helping young children fight off epilepsy and kept the episodes away.

The ketogenic diet needed to be used over the long-term, usually for two years or more, but helped children to not have to deal with the horrible effects of their seizures and helped them to reduce the amount of medication they needed to take.

Almost everyone is able to benefit from the use of the ketogenic diet.

It is different compared to some of the other diet plans that are available on the market, but this is part of what makes it so successful compared to the other diet plans.

When you are ready to start losing weight and improving many other aspects of your health, then make sure to try out the ketogenic diet to help you out.

Chapter 3: The Side Effects of the Ketogenic Diet

Before you get started with the ketogenic diet, it is important to know that there are some side effects or using and practicing the ketogenic diet.

These side effects are not horrible side effects like what you may be used to with common medications, but it is still a good idea to know what to expect when you are getting started on this new diet plan.

Some of the side effects that you may encounter when you are on the ketogenic diet are:

Dizziness or Headaches

One of the first side effects that you may experience when you get started with the ketogenic diet includes dizziness and headaches.

Dizziness and headaches are really prevalent in those individuals who for a very long time consumed a lot of caffeine and sugar before starting the ketogenic diet.

Both caffeine and sugar are highly addictive and if you go cold turkey on them, you may have a few side effects during the beginning process of the ketogenic diet.

You may introduce a little caffeine or sugar later on in the ketogenic diet plan if you want, but for those individuals who experience having a lot of trouble starting this diet plan or who really are addicted to caffeine and sugar, it is best to cut them out completely.

The good news is that the symptoms of withdrawal are only going to last for a few days and they really are not that severe.

You may feel a little anxious or upset because you will crave the caffeine and sugars that you are trying to eliminate from your diet.

However, if you are able to overcome your cravings for caffeine and sugar during the initial process of the ketogenic diet, you will break the addictions and you will not feel so reliant on consuming them as much.

One thing that you may decide to try is to slowly cut out your sugar and caffeine intake before you go on the ketogenic diet.

This will help you to not have to deal with these withdrawal symptoms as much. This can make things easier since you will already be dealing with feeling tired as your body gets used to the fats instead of the carbs.

If you are thinking about going on the ketogenic diet, consider cutting down on the sugars and caffeine for at least a few weeks ahead of time and you will not have to deal with the headaches or the dizziness as much when you begin.

Leg Cramps

Some of those who decide to go on the ketogenic diet will complain of dealing with leg cramps, especially when they are trying to go to bed at night.

This is common when you are in the early phase of the ketogenic diet.

This is a big problem for those users who are not paying attention to their micronutrients on this diet plan and who are not taking in enough potassium on this diet plan.

There are a few things that you are able to do to make sure you are getting enough potassium.

You can first work to try and eat plenty of foods with healthy amounts of potassium in them.

If you are having trouble doing this, you may decide to take a supplement that has potassium inside of it.

Many beginners decide to take a potassium supplement to help prevent leg cramps because keeping track of the macronutrients and the micronutrients for good health can be difficult.

However, you need to work towards not depending on supplements and instead eat real foods that will provide you with all the nutrients your body needs without taking any supplements.

Constipation

If you are not watching your micronutrients when you are on the ketogenic diet, you may deal with the issue of constipation.

This can be really uncomfortable for most people to deal with and can make sticking with the ketogenic diet a bit difficult.

However, the solution to this problem is pretty simple.

To ensure that you are not going to deal with constipation on the ketogenic diet plan, make sure that the majority of carbs that you decide to eat come from healthy green vegetables, which are full of fiber.

You also need to drink a lot of water on this diet plan because water has been shown to combat and prevent constipation.

For those individuals who maybe are already dealing with constipation, you may try a laxative to help you out.

Bad Breath

Another side effect that you may need to deal with on the ketogenic diet is bad breath.

While on the ketogenic diet plan, the body is going to burn up fat so that you can use this fat as energy.

This is the process of ketosis and will help you to burn through fat in your diet and the fat that is sitting around your body.

Unfortunately, the ketones (burning fat used as energy) that are released in this process will leave you with bad breath and make your urine smell bad.

The smell is going to be a little bit different than you may experience when after eating smelly food or by those individuals who suffer from halitosis (bad breath resulting from health problems).

Some people even compare it to a fruity candy smell instead, but if you do not want your breath to smell at all, then it is important to find a few ways to get rid of the bad breath.

Chewing on some gum without sugar, using mouthwash, or chewing on parsley or mint can help to get rid of this smell while keeping you on the ketogenic diet.

Feeling Tired

There are many people who will get started on the ketogenic diet who claim they feel tired.

They get going on this plan and are excited about all the big promises of more energy when they eat more healthy fats and fewer carbs.

Then they start on this diet and the first few days or in the first week they will begin to feel really tired almost like they just don't have enough energy to get things done.

This is completely normal on the ketogenic diet and it is important to know that these energy lacking feelings are going to fade away pretty soon.

The reason that you feel so tired when you start the ketogenic diet is that the body basically doesn't have any fuel for energy.

Sure, you are taking in healthy foods and providing it with fuel, but the body is used to relying on carbs and doesn't know what it should do when you take the majority of those carbs away.

So, the body is basically searching around hoping that you will eat and take in the carbs that it needs for easy energy access.

When you don't eat carbs or consume enough carbs your body is basically working on very little to no energy for a little while.

The good news is that feeling tired is not going to last for a very long time. For most people, it takes less than a week for the body to start recognizing the fat as a good source of energy and it will switch over.

Once the body starts to realize that it can use fat for energy instead of carbs, you will start to notice a big change.

Your energy will come back in a big way and you will feel amazing in no time.

You will be able to keep going all day long, even with fewer calories, and will ensure that you feel great about this diet plan.

As you can see, none of these side effects are life-threatening or that big of a deal when it comes to the ketogenic diet.

These side effects can make you a little bit uncomfortable and may not be the most pleasant when you are dealing with bad breath and feeling tired.

However, these side effects will usually not last for a long time and once your body adjusts to the ketogenic diet plan, you will not have to worry about them any longer.

Chapter 4: Who Can Safely Go on the Ketogenic Diet?

In most cases, following the ketogenic diet is a great experience. There are so many great health benefits that you will be able to enjoy when it comes to the ketogenic diet.

Many people choose to go on the ketogenic diet because they are tired of not being able to lose weight or fight off all that excess fat that has been hanging around their body for a long time.

But weight loss is not the only reason that you may choose to go on the ketogenic diet. If you have been fighting diabetes and its side effects for some time, reducing the number of carbs and the glucose it produces can help combat this health issue.

If you are worried about your high cholesterol levels and high blood pressure, simply practicing and following the ketogenic diet plan can help you to reduce your risks with these health issues as well.

Even younger children who have been dealing with epilepsy and those children with other neurological conditions may be able to benefit with the help of the ketogenic diet.

The children may be able to reduce some of the symptoms that they are dealing with and some have even been able to no longer need to use the medication they are on when they accurately follow the ketogenic diet plan.

Anyone who is dealing with health diseases or wants to lose weight or just simply wants to live a healthier lifestyle will be able to discover that the ketogenic diet is a good tool to help them out.

It doesn't matter if you are a man or a woman, the ketogenic diet is the right option to help anyone.

Who Shouldn't Use the Ketogenic Diet?

There are so many people who are able to use the ketogenic diet. The ketogenic diet has a lot of benefits and it can help you to lose weight, fight off many health concerns, and help you to feel amazing in no time.

However, there are certain groups of people who should avoid and not practice the ketogenic diet.

Practicing the ketogenic diet plan can be detrimental to the health of some people and even make them feel sick.

Some of those individuals who should avoid the ketogenic diet are:

- Children and teenagers
- Women who are pregnant and breastfeeding
- Women with irregular menstrual cycles
- People that have issues with their thyroid glands
- People that suffer from adrenal fatigue
- High-level athletes who need carbs to help them function better

These groups of people will often not do as well with the ketogenic diet.

This is because they need special dietary requirements that are eliminated from their diet when they follow the ketogenic diet.

For example, a pregnant or nursing mother needs to take in carbs to help her baby to grow and eliminating these completely can result in a nutrient deficiency for the baby.

Teenagers and children often need some of the glucose that is found in carbs, or they need higher carb content from fruits and vegetables than the ketogenic diet allows.

This does not mean that these groups of people can't take some advice from the ketogenic diet to help them stay healthy.

For example, teenagers or pregnant women may choose to limit their carbs a bit, but not to the fifty grams a day that is recommended by the ketogenic diet.

Instead, teenagers or pregnant women can instead stick to eating healthy carbs like fruits and vegetables while reducing their intake of unhealthy carbs like the bread and pastas that they normally eat.

Teenagers or pregnant women can also consider increasing their healthy fat intake and eating good amounts of protein each day.

So basically, some of these groups of people can follow some of the principles of the ketogenic diet without following or practicing so many of the restrictions the actual diet requires.

If you fall into one of the groups above, it may be a good idea to talk to your doctor before attempting to go on this diet plan.

This will help you to determine if you really need the ketogenic diet and if it is actually a healthy option for you, especially if you are in one of the groups above.

Chapter 5: The Ketogenic Diet and Exercise

It is important to understand how exercise and your fitness performance can be affected by the ketogenic diet.

It is also important to understand that maybe your exercise routine/plan/goals may need to be changed a little bit as a result of practicing the ketogenic diet.

However, you will still see some great results from your fitness workouts while practicing the ketogenic diet.

In additional, habitual exercise combined with the ketogenic diet will help you to lose weight and fat faster than ever.

You may also need to add a few extra carbs to your diet in order to have the right amount of energy for achieving your health and fitness goals.

With the ketogenic diet, you are greatly reducing the number of carbs that you are consuming and since many athletes require carbs to help them stay energetic, you may be curious to know how this is going to affect your body when you enter ketosis.

You will need to keep a few things in mind when you get started on the ketogenic diet when it comes to exercising, but it is just fine to exercise on this diet and all the health benefits definitely make it worth your time.

First, we need to understand that the traditional view on weight loss, the idea that you just need to eat less and exercise for a longer period of time (while getting plenty of cardio in as well) is advice that is outdated and just won't work with the ketogenic diet.

To really lose weight and get that leaner frame that you have been looking for, the foods that you eat while on the ketogenic diet are what matter the most.

Eating recommended foods on the ketogenic diet like meats, seafood, and dairy are great ways to begin the ketogenic diet.

The most important thing you can do for weight loss and maintaining your energy levels is to pay attention to how well and how disciplined you are to following the ketogenic diet.

If you are able to remain in a steady state of ketosis, rather than coming in and out of it because you can't keep your carbs steady or low, you will see some amazing results.

Before you decide to start doing more and more of your regular physical exercise activities while on the ketogenic diet, make sure that you understand when your body is in ketosis as well as spend some time testing your ketone levels.

However, once you get used to how the ketogenic diet works, adding in exercise can provide you with a lot of good benefits to your health.

Physical exercise like strength training and lifting weights will help to make your bones stronger as well as build muscle and make you have that lean look you want.

In addition, physical exercise like strength training and lifting weights is also great for the heart.

And as long as you are taking in nutrients properly on the ketogenic diet, physical exercise can easily fit in with your new diet plan.

Just remember that when you are exercising while on the ketogenic diet, make sure to stay healthy, make sure your energy levels are good and don't harm yourself while practicing the ketogenic diet.

Why Should I Exercise on the Ketogenic Diet?

After learning a bit more about ketosis and how the body needs higher levels of carbs in order to properly perform the activities that you would like, you may think that ketosis is not the best for long-term exercise.

However, exercising while on the ketogenic diet actually provides the user with many benefits including:

- In one study, ultra-endurance athletes were asked to do a three-hour run.

  Those who ate a low carb diet for about twenty months on average had up to three times the fat burn compared to the athletes who followed a high-carb diet.

  Both of these groups were able to replenish the same amount of muscle glycogen when done.

- Studies have shown that ketosis can help to prevent fatigue in people who exercise for long periods of time.

  For example, people that strength train for 1 or 2 hours or people who do cardio exercise activities such as running have sufficient energy to complete their long workouts.

- Ketosis is great for helping to maintain your blood glucose levels, whether you are considered obese or not.

- With the help of keto-adaption (which we will talk about later on), low-carb ketogenic dieters are actually better able to perform various activities, even while taking in fewer carbs over time.

- You receive all the regular benefits of exercise. In addition to the benefits listed above, those individuals who are on the ketogenic diet are able to receive all the same benefits that they would receive on any other diet while working out.

  However, the main difference between the ketogenic diet and other diets is that the ketogenic diet uses fat as energy instead of carbs.

  Keep this in mind, exercising while on the ketogenic diet will help you to be in a better mood, lose weight, see fat loss, control your blood sugar levels, reduce blood pressure, and so much more.

  Everyone should consider starting on their own workout program and combining it with the ketogenic diet.

  It is important to state that having a good mixture of different exercises, from flexibility to strength training and some lower-intensity aerobics or cardio exercises, will help you to make the whole body strong and will prevent injuries along the way.

While you may need to take a little bit of time off from working out when you first get started with the ketogenic diet to help you adjust, most people are able to successfully work out while practicing the ketogenic diet.

By making a few adjustments to your ketogenic lifestyle and by watching how many carbs you eat as well as when you consume your carbs will make all the difference in the results that you see when it comes to achieving your weight loss goals.

Types of Exercises to do While on the Ketogenic Diet

Your nutritional needs are going to vary based on the exercise or exercises that you want to perform. But generally, you will be able to divide up exercises into four group.

These four groups of exercises include stability training, flexibility training, anaerobic exercises, and aerobic exercises.

Let's take a look at how each of these can work with the ketogenic diet:

- **Aerobic exercise:** Aerobic exercise is typically known as cardio (swimming, running, cycling) and it will be any activity that gets the heart up and running for more than three minutes.

  As a result, your body may require more carbs while practicing the ketogenic diet.

  If you do cardio exercises that are steady-state and lower in intensity like walking you are going to be concentrating on fat burning, which makes it a great exercise for the ketogenic diet.

- **Anaerobic exercise:** This type of exercise is going to have short bursts of energy throughout an exercise session, such as HIIT, powerlifting or explosive exercises.

If you plan to do anaerobic exercises, you may need to take in more carbs because anaerobic exercises require a lot more carbs as their primary fuel source.

Make sure that when you combine anaerobic exercises with the ketogenic diet that you consume just a little more carbs just for the sake of making sure you have the necessary energy to complete your physical workouts.

- **Flexibility training:** It is a good idea to add some flexibility exercises to your fitness routine.

  Flexibility training can be helpful for stretching out the muscles, improving your range of motion, and supporting the joints.

  Flexibility training is often used to help prevent injuries from some of the other workouts that you may do.

  Some examples of flexibility training are Yoga and just simple stretching exercises.

  Flexibility training does not require a lot of carbs. As a result, the ketogenic diet is perfect for people that do Yoga or simple stretching exercises.

- **Stability exercises:** Stability exercises are exercises that work on your core or abdominal (abs) muscles as well as help improve your balance.

  Stability exercises are good for helping control your body's movements, strengthen the muscles in the body, and can even improve your body's alignment.

Stability exercises do not require a lot of carbs.

As a result, the ketogenic diet is perfect for people that practice stability exercises.

Keep this in mind when you are exercising while practicing the ketogenic diet:

"Mix up your workouts as much as possible. Do a combination of all four types of exercises and or training mentioned above for the purpose of developing the type of body that you want.

At the same time always monitor your energy levels to make sure you are consuming just enough carbs while practicing the ketogenic diet.

If at any moment you are feeling too tired to complete your workout routine simply stop exercising, monitor your energy levels and see if you need to increase your carbs intake. Safety first."

It is important to state that as you practice the ketogenic diet and you reach ketosis, the intensity of your exercise workouts is going to matter quite a bit.

When you do low-intensity workouts like walking or Yoga, the body will rely more on fat as its energy source, so these workouts are the best for those on the ketogenic diet.

The high-intensity aerobic exercises, like jogging and running, and anaerobic exercises, like powerlifting and sprinting, are going to rely more on carbs as an energy source and are not the best exercises to do while practicing the ketogenic diet.

Just keep in mind that if you are going to do high-intensity exercises you may need to add some more carbs to your diet.

Picking a Targeted Ketogenic Diet (Variations)

So far, we have just been talking about the basic ketogenic diet. This is a great diet if you are looking to get started and you don't plan to do really intense workouts.

The ketogenic diet will often work for regular exercise and for a little bit of low-intensity activities as well.

But if you are planning on doing activities that are more intense, or you plan to exercise or workout more than three days out of the week to help with weight and fat loss, then it is time to consider a targeted ketogenic diet variation.

A targeted ketogenic diet variation will help you to adjust your diet so that you get enough carbs to help you achieve your fitness goals as well as keep you in ketosis.

Those higher intensity workouts, like lots of weightlifting and sprinting are not going to do well with the regular ketogenic diet so having a targeted ketogenic diet variation will help you get the results that you would like.

These targeted ketogenic diet variations will allow you to have some more carbs during the day so that you can maintain your activity levels.

This does not mean that you can go out and enjoy as many sodas and baked goods as you like.

You still need to get your carbs from keto approved foods, like fruits and vegetables, but you are allowed to increase your healthy carb intake.

A good thing to remember is that you should eat about 15 to 30 grams of fast acting carbs (which includes options like fruit) about twenty minutes before and after your workout.

This helps your muscles to get the glycogen that they need to do well during training and so that your muscles can recover.

Eating during that time period will ensure that the carbs are used for the workout, so you won't leave ketosis at all.

Options or Variations of the Ketogenic Diet

There are a few options for the ketogenic diet that you can pick based on the amount of physical activity that you plan to do.

The different ketogenic diet variations that you can choose from include:

- **The standard ketogenic diet:** With this diet option you will keep your total carb count between 20 to 50 grams each day.

- **The targeted ketogenic diet:** With this diet option, you will stick with the 20 to 50 grams of carbs each day. But you will plan out when you eat these carbs.

  You will want to get the majority, if not all, of these carbs about an hour or less before you do your exercise. This is the best option for athletes who like to do high-intensity activities like weightlifting, sprinting, CrossFit, etc.,

- **The cyclical ketogenic diet:** For this one, you will cut your carbs down to almost nothing for a few days.

And then on the days that you want to do a higher-intensity workout, you will eat higher-carbs on that day. This should even out for the right amount of carbs throughout the week.

Depending on the exercises that you are doing you may find that the carb content is too low, and you are not taking in enough carbs to keep up with your activity levels.

If you want to know if you are in a state of ketosis, you can simply purchase some test strips at the local pharmacy that will help you to know whether you are in ketosis or not.

You may also be able to increase your carb intake a little bit and still remain in the state of ketosis.

However, it is important to be careful when you slightly increase your carbs intake because it is really easy to jump out of ketosis.

In addition, if you do jump out of ketosis then you will lose the benefits of the ketogenic diet plan if you aren't closely monitoring how many carbs you consume.

The good news is that most people are able to adapt to eating lower-carb diets and using fat to help them get the fuel that they need.

This may take a few weeks and you may not be as strong for those first few weeks as the body adjusts. However, the longer you remain on the ketogenic diet, the more the body can adapt to this diet plan.

After practicing the ketogenic diet for a while, your body will become more efficient at burning the fat and using up the ketones that are in the body.

With enough physical exercise and after a while of being on the ketogenic diet, you will be able to see some amazing results with your body as well as achieve whatever fitness goals you plan to achieve.

Chapter 6: What Should I Eat on the Ketogenic Diet?

One question that a lot of people will ask when getting started on the ketogenic diet is what they are allowed to eat.

Working with the right macronutrients is one of the most important parts of the ketogenic diet. You must make sure that you are eating plenty of healthy fats and low carbs so that you can stay in ketosis.

Actually, eating plenty of healthy fats and low carbs is going to be one of the most important things that you concentrate on when it comes to the ketogenic diet.

However, as long as the foods that you eat fit into these macronutrients, and you are getting plenty of vitamins and minerals from the fruits and vegetables you choose to eat, you will lose weight.

Before we look at the specific foods that you are able to eat on the ketogenic diet let's take a look at the macronutrients.

This is really important and will ensure that you are eating enough fats to stay energetic as well as keeping the carbs low enough so that you don't kick yourself out of ketosis.

Also, don't forget that it is important to eat healthy sources of protein rich foods so that you can keep your muscles big and strong.

First, let's take a look at the fats that you need to eat. It is recommended that you get somewhere between 70 to 75 percent of your daily calories from healthy fats.

You must make sure that these are healthy fats. Going to the local fast food restaurant and eating a big burger and fries will not count because these are bad fats that will not help out with the ketogenic diet.

Instead, eating healthy fats like olive oil, fats from dairy products, and fats that come in healthy protein sources are much better options.

You will also need to eat moderate amounts of protein as well. You will need between 15 and 20 percent of your daily calories from protein.

This helps to keep the muscles as strong as possible and can be especially important if you are someone who likes to work out a lot and wants to build muscle with the ketogenic diet plan. Stick with options like healthy fish, chicken, turkey, and ground beef.

And finally, most people will want to keep their carb intake down to five percent or lower. If you are really into weight lifting, you can sometimes go up to ten percent.

But, before you increase your carbs intake, make sure that you experiment and see if you are really in ketosis with the higher amount of carbs or not.

Remember, when choosing carbs to eat stick with healthy options like fruits and vegetables that will help to keep you feeling full.

In addition, eating healthy carbs like fruits and vegetables will give your body the vitamins and nutrients that your body needs.

If you are able to stick with these macronutrients, you will see great results with the ketogenic diet.

It will take some time to get used to which foods will fit into this diet plan, but once you get used to it, losing weight and fat will be easier than ever before.

Foods to Eat on the Ketogenic Diet

Sticking with the macronutrients that we talked about above is one of the most important things that you can do on this diet plan.

But putting this into a meal plan can be difficult when you first get started.

Some of the foods that you are able to enjoy when following the ketogenic diet include:

- **Meat:** There are many different types of meat that you can enjoy, and this will provide you with the protein and some of the fats that you need.

You can choose from options like fish, lamb, veal, pork, venison, chicken, quail, duck, and shellfish.

With chicken, make sure that you leave the skin on to help increase the fat content, but do not bread or batter any poultry that you eat.

Make sure that you do not eat any processed meats, though. If choosing canned fish options, make sure that the preservation method does not use any added sugar.

- **Eggs:** Many meals on the ketogenic diet will require you to eat eggs for the purpose of consuming both protein and healthy fat.

Because eggs have lots of healthy protein and fats, they can be eaten for breakfast, lunch or dinner.

- **Cheese:** For the most part, cheese is a good food to eat while on the ketogenic diet. There are a few carbs found in the different varieties of cheese, so make sure to read the labels carefully and then count the carbs before you eat them.

  Some cheese may push you over your daily required carbs intake so make sure you keep track of other carbs you have eaten that day.

- **Vegetables:** Vegetables will contain most of the carbs that you are going to eat but try to keep this to a minimum.

  You should go with the green and leafy options because these are lower in carbs so options like lettuce, cabbage, kale, and watercress are great.

  You can also go with options like bean sprouts, cucumber, celery, broccoli, and asparagus.

- **Fruits:** You can enjoy some fruits on the ketogenic diet, but you need to be careful about which ones you eat.

  Some fruits can be higher in carbs compared to some of the other food options on the list and if you eat too many fruits, you will end up going over your daily required carbs intake.

  If you choose to add some fruits to your diet, carefully watch your portions and avoid going over on the carb content.

One recommended fruit is the avocado. The avocado is a good source of healthy fat so try to make the avocado part of your ketogenic diet meal plan.

- **Nuts:** Nuts are a good source of healthy fats and protein so they are fine to eat as long as you eat them in moderation as a type of dessert or as a snack. Some recommended nuts are walnuts.

- **Cream, butter, and oils** are usually fine because they provide you with some healthy sources of fat.

- **Dry spices** and **fresh herbs** are great for the ketogenic diet. Dry spices and fresh herbs will help you to get some flavoring in your meals without adding in any extra carbs.

As you can see, while you do need to be careful with the macronutrients that you are consuming on the ketogenic diet, there are still some options that you can go with to eat great meals.

Mix and match some of the options that were mentioned above, and you will get tasty meals that are easy to make and will help you to lose weight without feeling hungry.

Foods to Avoid on the Ketogenic Diet

For the most part, if the foods are not listed in the section above, you should not consume them on the ketogenic diet.

Consuming foods that are not recommended for the ketogenic diet can add in too many bad fats, bad carbs, and sugars than your body does not need.

In addition, consuming foods that are not recommended for the ketogenic diet may kick you out of your ketosis state.

Keep in mind that you do not want to work hard to get into ketosis and then end up cheating yourself and getting kicked out of ketosis because you consumed foods that are not recommended for the ketogenic diet.

Some of the foods that you will need to avoid on the ketogenic diet are:

- **Bread and pasta:** Bread and pasta may seem healthy, but just a small serving can put you over your required daily carb intake.

  There are healthier alternatives, such as keto bread or using vegetables to make noodles, so you can still enjoy some of your favorite meals without having to worry about eating too many carbs.

- **Baked goods:** In between the excess carbs and sugars that are inside most baked goods, it is no wonder that baked goods are not allowed on the ketogenic diet.

  It is best to stick with eating a piece of fruit (especially if you can find one that is lower in carbs) for your snack rather than eating any of the baked goods that are available.

- **Processed frozen foods/meals:** Anything that you can find in the freezer section of your grocery store should be avoided.

  These may seem healthy, but the preservatives and carbs are extremely high and will kick you out of ketosis.

It is best to just leave everything that is in the freezer section alone and stick with fresh and whole foods instead.

- **Sodas:** Some people choose to drink diet sodas when they are on the ketogenic and diet sodas are allowed. However, you should avoid regular sodas because of all the sugar that is inside of them.

- **Fast foods:** While you are on the ketogenic diet, you need to avoid going out to eat.

  Fast foods are full of way too many carbs and bad fats and will instantly take you out of ketosis without much effort. Avoid fast foods and just cook your meals at home instead.

- **Deli meats:** Deli meats may seem like a good option to get your protein, but in reality, they are mostly processed and full of lots of carbs.

  It is best to avoid deli meats as much as possible and focus your time and energy on eating healthier proteins and carbs.

It is important that you eat the right foods when it comes to the ketogenic diet.

There are some other diet plans that will allow you to cheat on occasion, but when you cheat on the ketogenic diet, you lose all of your weight loss benefits.

If you would like to stay in ketosis and really lose weight, then make sure to avoid the foods mentioned above and you will see great results with the ketogenic diet.

Chapter 7: Simple Meal Plans for the Ketogenic Diet

One of the hardest things that many beginners have trouble with is figuring out what they need to eat on the ketogenic diet.

While they may understand how the macronutrients are supposed to work on the diet, they are worried about how to plan out their meals and how to make it work well for them.

Coming up with ideas for your ketogenic meal plans is one of the best things that you can do because it outlines what you need to eat for the whole week or longer if you like.

Now, we are going to look at a simple one-week meal plan that you can follow to get started on the ketogenic diet and see amazing results in no time.

Monday
Breakfast: Scrambled Eggs
Lunch: Keto Asian Salad
Dinner: Pesto Chicken Casserole

Tuesday
Breakfast: Cheese Roll-ups
Lunch: Egg Omelet
Dinner: Meat Pie

Wednesday

Breakfast:	Frittata with Spinach
Lunch:	Chicken Soup (No Noodle)
Dinner:	Carbonara

Thursday

Breakfast:	Dairy Free Latte
Lunch:	Avocado and Goat Cheese Salad
Dinner:	Keto Pizza

Friday

Breakfast:	Mushroom Omelet
Lunch:	Smoked Salmon
Dinner:	Keto Tacos

Saturday

Breakfast:	Baked Bacon Omelet
Lunch:	Keto Quesadillas
Dinner:	Asian Stir-Fry

Sunday

Breakfast:	Berry Pancakes
Lunch:	Italian Keto Plate
Dinner:	Pork Chops

Keto Recipes

Recipe #1
Scrambled Eggs with Spinach
What's in it?

- Some salt
- Pepper

- Butter (1 oz.)
- Eggs (2)
- Spinach

How's it done?

Whisk together the eggs while adding the pepper and salt.

Add some butter to a skillet and let it warm up. When the butter is hot, pour the eggs and let them cook.

After two minutes, the eggs should be creamy. Add some spinach to your eggs and you can finish scrambling and enjoy!

Keto Recipe #2
Pesto Chicken Casserole
What's in it?

- Peppers
- Some salt
- Chopped garlic cloves (1)
- Diced feta cheese (8 oz.)
- Pitted olives (8 Tbsp.)
- Heavy whip cream (1.5 cups)
- Green pesto (3 oz.)
- Butter (2 oz.)
- Chicken thighs (1.5 lbs.)
- Leafy greens (5.3 oz.)
- Olive oil (4 Tbsp.)

How's it done?

1. Allow the oven to heat up to 400 degrees. While the oven is heating up, cut up the chicken thighs into pieces and season them with pepper and salt.

2. Add the chicken to a skillet and fry them with some butter to make them nice and brown.

3. In another bowl, mix together the heavy cream and the pesto. Place the chicken pieces into a prepared baking dish.

4. Top the chicken with the pesto, garlic, feta cheese, and olives. Place everything into the oven to bake.

5. After 30 minutes, the dish is done and ready to eat.

Keto Recipe #3
Cheese Roll-Ups
What's in it?
- Butter (2 oz.)
- Cheddar cheese (8 oz.)

How's it done?

1. Take the cheese slices onto a cutting board. Slice the butter with a cheese slicer so you end up with thin slices.

2. Cover each of these slices with some butter before rolling them up and then serve and eat.

Keto Recipe #4
Chicken Soup
What's in it?

- Sliced green cabbage (2 cups)
- Shredded chicken (1.5 lbs.)
- Carrot (1)
- Chicken broth (8 cups)
- Pepper (.25 tsp.)
- Salt (1 tsp.)
- Parsley (2 tsp.)
- Minced onion (2 Tbsp.)
- Garlic cloves (2)
- Mushrooms, sliced (6 oz.)
- Celery stalks (2)
- Butter (4 oz.)

How's it done?

1. Start this out by melting the butter in a pot. Slice up the mushrooms and the celery into small pieces.

2. Add these to a pot along with the garlic and dried onion and cook for a few minutes.

3. After this time, add the pepper, salt, parsley, carrot, and broth. Let it all simmer until they become tender.

4. Add the cabbage and the chicken and cook for about 12 more minutes so the noodles are tender before serving.

Keto Recipe #5
Keto Pizza
What's in it?

- *Crust*
- Shredded cheese (6 oz.)
- Eggs (4)
- *Toppings*
- Salt
- Pepper
- Olive oil (4 Tbsp.)
- Leafy greens (5.5 oz.)
- Olives
- Pepperoni (1.75 oz.)
- Shredded cheese (4.25 oz.)
- Dried oregano (1 tsp.)
- Tomato paste (3 Tbsp.)

How's it done?

1. Allow the oven to heat up to 400 degrees. While the oven warms up, take out a bowl and beat the cheese and eggs together to make the crust. Spread this out on a prepared baking sheet, making one large pizza or two small pizzas.

2. Place the pizza(s) in the oven to bake. After 15 minutes, the crust will be golden and you can take the pizza(s) out of the oven.

3. Allow the temperature of your oven to get to 450 degrees. Spread out the tomato paste on your crust and add on the rest of the toppings.

4. Place the pizza(s) back into the oven for a bit and after ten minutes, the pizza(s) should be ready. Serve with some leafy green vegetables and enjoy.

Keto Recipe #6
Smoked Salmon
What's in it?
- Pepper
- Salt
- Lime (1/2)
- Olive oil (1 Tbsp.)
- Baby spinach (2 oz.)
- Mayo (1 cup)
- Smoked salmon (.75 lbs.)

How's it done?

1. To start, bring out a plate and put the lime wedge, spinach, salmon and some mayo all on one plate.

2. Drizzle a bit of oil on top of the spinach before seasoning with the pepper and the salt. Serve this right away and eat.

Keto Recipe #7

Mushroom Omelet
What's in it?
- Pepper
- Salt
- Mushrooms (3)
- Yellow onion (1/3)

- Shredded cheese (1 oz.)
- Butter (1 oz.)
- Eggs (3)

How's it done?

1. To start this recipe, bring out a mixing bowl and crack the eggs inside. Season the eggs with pepper and salt and continue whisking to make them frothy.

2. Melt some butter in a skillet and then when it is warm, add the egg mixture.

3. When you notice this omelet is firming but is still a bit raw, add the onion, mushrooms, and cheese to the top.

4. Use a spatula to ease around the edges of your omelet so you can fold it in half. Take off the heat and serve.

Keto Recipe #8
Keto Quesadillas
What's in it?
- *Tortillas*
- Salt (1/2 tsp.)
- Coconut flour (1 Tbsp.)
- Ground psyllium husk powder (1.5 tsp.)
- Cream cheese (6 oz.)
- Egg whites (2)
- Eggs (2)
- *Filling*
- Olive oil (1 Tbsp.)
- Leafy greens (1 oz.)

- Shredded cheese (5 oz.)

How's it done?

1. Allow the oven to heat up to 400 degrees. While the oven is heating up, beat together your egg whites and eggs for a few minutes to make them fluffy. Add the cream cheese to your eggs and mix until they are nice and smooth.

2. In another bowl, whisk together the coconut flour, psyllium husk powder, and salt. Next, add these ingredients to your bowl of eggs and cream cheese a little at a time.

3. When the batter is combined, let it sit for a bit so it becomes thick like pancake batter.

4. Place two baking sheets on the counter and add parchment paper. Pour three circles of the dough on each sheet and spread into thin rounds.

5. Next, place the two sheets of dough into the oven and let the dough cook for a bit. After five minutes, you can take the tortillas out.

6. When the tortillas have cooled down, place them onto a cutting board and add some cheese on the tortillas. Also, add on some leafy green vegetables and the rest of the cheese on the tortilla and then top it with a second tortilla.

7. Take out a skillet and add in some oil. Fry each of the quesadillas in the skillet for a bit on each side, letting the cheese melt.

8. After this is done, cut up the quesadillas and then serve and eat.

Keto Recipe #9
Asian Stir-Fry
What's in it?

- Sesame oil (1 Tbsp.)
- Ginger (1 Tbsp.)
- Chili flakes (1 tsp)
- Sliced scallions (3)
- Garlic cloves (2)
- White wine vinegar (1 Tbsp.)
- Pepper (.25 tsp. or 1/4 tsp.)
- Onion powder (1 tsp.)
- Salt (1 tsp.)
- Ground beef (1.5 lbs.)
- Butter (5.5 oz.)
- Green cabbage (1.66 lbs.)
- *Wasabi Mayo*
- Wasabi paste (1 Tbsp.)
- Mayonnaise (1 cup)

How's it done?

1. Shred up the cabbage with your food processor. Add some butter to a frying pan and then fry your cabbage for a few minutes.

2. Add the vinegar and spices and cook for a few more minutes before putting the cabbage in a bowl.

3. Melt the remainder of the butter before adding the ginger, chili flakes, and garlic and then let it cook. Add the meat and let it get brown all the way through.

4. Add the cabbage and the scallions to this mixture and stir to make it hot. Top with sesame oil, pepper, and salt.

5. Before serving, mix the ingredients together with the mayonnaise. Serve this stir-fry with some of the wasabi mayo on top.

Keto Recipe #10
Keto Pancakes
What's in it?

- Butter (2 oz.)
- Ground psyllium husk powder (1 Tbsp.)
- Cottage cheese (7 oz.)
- Eggs (4)
- *Toppings Below*
- Whipping cream (1 cup)
- Fresh berries (8 Tbsp.)

How's it done?

1. To start this recipe, take out a bowl and blend all the batter ingredients together. Set the bowl to the side and let it expand for at least five minutes.

2. When you are ready, heat up a bit of the oil in a pan. Add some of the batter to the pan and let the batter cook for three minutes on both sides. Make sure to flip the batter (pancake) carefully.

3. Turn off the heat when the pancake is done and serve with the heavy cream and the berries of your choice before enjoying your meal.

Chapter 8: The Ketogenic Diet vs. Intermittent Fasting

The ketogenic diet can be a very effective diet plan.

If you are able to eat the right foods and closely monitor your macronutrients, you will enter into ketosis and see big results.

Still, some people hit a rut with their weight loss goals or simply need to do even more to help improve their overall health.

As a result, working with just the ketogenic diet may not be enough for some people. One diet alternative that people can choose to practice is called intermittent fasting.

What is Intermittent Fasting?

Intermittent fasting is more of a lifestyle than a diet. Intermittent fasting is simply fasting or not eating food for a certain period of time.

Now that period of time of fasting or not eating food is usually between 12-16 hours. However, many people experience better results by fasting for 16 or more hours.

There are a lot of different variations when it comes to intermittent fasting, so you can choose the method that works the best for your schedule or for you to maintain for the long term.

Let's take a look at some of the basics of intermittent fasting so you can see how it will work well with the ketogenic diet.

The Intermittent Fasting Approach

There are actually a few different approaches that you can use when it comes to intermittent fasting.

Each intermittent fasting approach can be effective, and it is often based on what fits your schedule.

The most common approaches that you can use with intermittent fasting are:

- **Skipping meals:** With this option, you will skip over a meal or two so that you can induce some extra time for fasting.

  So, for example, skipping breakfast or simply not eating in the morning can be one intermittent fasting approach.

  Skipping breakfast is one of the most effective methods for practicing intermittent fasting simply because you are already fasting all night from you last meal (dinner).

  If you must eat breakfast every morning than maybe try to skip either lunch and simply eat dinner.

  The benefit of this intermittent fasting approach is that it allows you to experiment to see what works for you and your schedule.

- **Eating windows:** With this intermittent fasting approach, you are going to work on getting all of your macronutrients within a certain eating schedule.

For example, a person can have an eating window from 12:00 PM-7:00 PM. So, this means a person can eat from 12:00 PM – 7:00 PM.

So, while most people eat from when they get up until when they go to bed, a personal practicing this intermittent fasting approach will reduce their eating time to windows of four to eight hours depending on their work and lifestyle schedules.

For example, you can have an eating window from 8:00 AM – 4:00 PM. So, this means you can only eat between 8:00 AM – 4:00 PM.

So, within this eating window you can eat two or three small meals. This intermittent fasting approach is good because you can experiment to see what is convenient for your work and lifestyle schedules.

- **One to two-day cleanses:** With this intermittent fasting approach, you are going to put yourself on an extended fasting period.

  With one to two-day cleanses, you will simply avoid eating for one or two days. You can do one or two-day cleanses once or twice a week.

  Now this intermittent fasting approach will effectively reduce the number of calories that you consume resulting in great weight loss.

  Most people will find that it is hard to start out with a one or two day fast, which is why restricting your eating window or skipping meals are two of the best intermittent fasting approaches you can choose from.

Remember to experiment with intermittent fasting and try out different eating windows for a week or so to see what intermittent fasting approach works best for you.

How Does Intermittent Fasting Work?

While there are a few different options when it comes to choosing an intermittent fasting approach, you may wonder why it can be so effective.

The whole point of intermittent fasting is to simply eat food during a certain period of time.

Our bodies will only be able to take in so much food at once, so if we are only allowed to eat for a few hours during the day and then fast during the rest, we are limiting our calorie intake which results in weight loss.

During the fasting time, we are not allowed to eat at all. Our metabolism also seems to speed up as long as the fasting period is short, such as fasting for just eighteen hours rather than for a whole week or more.

So not only are we reducing the calories that we are able to consume because our bodies can't take in that much food at one time, we are also speeding up our metabolism at the same time.

Over time, your body is going to learn how to adjust to intermittent fasting.

In the beginning, intermittent fasting is going to be hard and you may feel hungry during the fasting period.

But if you can maintain your periods of fasting, the body will eventually adapt and you will be able to feel just fine without eating all day long.

In addition, maintaining your periods of fasting and keeping track of the food you eat will eventually become easier when you only have a few hours a day to eat.

It is important to state that when you are in a fasting state, the body is able to break down some of the extra fat that is being stored by your body.

Now if you include ketosis from the ketogenic diet, all of the excess fat that you have on your body will simply melt off in no time.

In addition, you will still have plenty of energy for all of your daily activities.

Ketosis actually mimics the fasting state because we take the glucose out of our bloodstream so that we can use fats as our main source of energy.

During your fast, the body is going to rely on those extra fat stores to help you to stay energized.

If you are doing intermittent fasting along with the ketogenic diet, you need to make sure that you really get the sufficient amount of fat content that the body needs so that the body can get the right amounts of energy that it needs.

It is important to state that when you combine both intermittent fasting and the ketogenic diet together, you will be able to burn through fat, lower your glucose levels, and see tremendous results in your overall health.

Intermittent fasting is not necessarily for weight loss, although it can help you to lose weight if you are prone to overeating throughout the day.

In addition, intermittent fasting can help you reduce your calorie intake resulting in weight loss.

When you combine intermittent fasting with the ketogenic diet, you are sure to see some tremendous weight loss results as well as an increase in your health benefits.

Are the Ketogenic Diet and Intermittent Fasting Similar?

There are a few similarities that you will find with the ketogenic diet and intermittent fasting.

Both are going to work to limit the amount of glucose in your diet so that the body will start to rely more on using fats for energy rather than carbs and sugars for energy.

This is an effective way to melt the fat off your body and help you to lose weight.

However, the methods that both use to help you reach this result are different. The ketogenic diet helps you to use fat as energy by changing up the macronutrients that you consume to cut out the carbs.

Intermittent fasting will help you to burn fat because you will be forced to reduce how many calories you are able to consume as a result of having a small eating window.

The ketogenic diet is an eating plan. With the ketogenic diet you have certain foods that you are able to consume, and you need to stick with eating those specific foods if you want to be on this diet plan.

On the other hand, intermittent fasting can be done with any type of diet plan. However, intermittent fasting will not be effective if you only eat junk food during your eating window.

But you can combine intermittent fasting with other diets such as the Mediterranean diet, or any other diet plan that you choose.

But when intermittent fasting is combined with the ketogenic diet, you are going to get some amazing weight loss results and your overall health will greatly improve.

Can I Use Intermittent Fasting and the Ketogenic Diet Together?

Yes, it is possible to use both intermittent fasting and the ketogenic diet together.

Keep in mind, intermittent fasting is more about fasting or not eating for a certain period of time each and every day and that period of time can be between 12-16 hours or more.

Now the ketogenic diet is more about the types of foods that you would eat each and every day specifically low carbs, a lot of healthy fats and moderate protein.

It is important to state that you do not have to go on an intermittent fasting diet in order to lose weight with the ketogenic diet.

It is already hard enough for many people to follow the ketogenic diet so combining both intermittent fasting and the ketogenic diet for weight loss is not required, but instead an option.

But for those people who would like to experiment and seek to achieve their weight loss goals and improve their overall health, then combining both intermittent fasting and the ketogenic diet is definitely a great idea.

With intermittent fasting, you will limit the hours that you are able to eat. Instead of allowing yourself to spread your meals and your snacks all throughout the day, you will limit your "eating window" to just a few hours a day.

With intermittent fasting, many people will choose to only eat between 10:00 AM - 6:00 PM and eat all of their macronutrients during this time period.

Others will do a whole day of fasting once or twice a week where they are not allowed to eat at all for one full day.

When people do a full day of fasting they try to consume all of their nutrients on the other days of the week in order to have sufficient energy for their one full day of fasting.

Just keep in mind that the point of intermittent fasting is that you are limiting the amount of time that you are able to eat which forces you to eat fewer calories which results in weight loss.

Now if you ever feel like you hit a plateau with your weight loss goals while on the ketogenic diet, simply consider combining the ketogenic diet with intermittent fasting.

Combining both the ketogenic diet and intermittent fasting will definitely "shock" the body and you will also benefit greatly by burning more fat and achieving your weight loss goals.

When you combine intermittent fasting with the ketogenic diet, you must remember to stick with the macronutrients that we discussed above that are approved for the ketogenic diet.

So, you will still stick with a high fat, moderate protein, and low carb diet plan even while intermittent fasting.

You will just need to be more careful about the times you eat those macronutrients, but otherwise, you can follow the ketogenic diet exactly the same.

If you want to get some of the benefits that come with intermittent fasting or you want to increase your weight loss, then combining intermittent fasting with the ketogenic diet can be very effective.

You can experiment with the different types of intermittent fasting variations that are available to see which one fits into your schedule and works best for you.

Of course, if you find the ketogenic diet is effective enough or adding in intermittent fasting is too difficult, you can always just stay with the ketogenic diet on its own and still see some amazing results.

Conclusion

Thank you for making it through the end of this book.

I hope the book was educational, informative and able to provide you with all of the tools you need to achieve your health and weight loss goals or whatever they may be.

The next step is to get started with the ketogenic diet.

This is one of the most effective diet plans that is available for helping you to lose weight.

While you will need to get used to some of the dietary changes that are unusual compared to other traditional diet plans, the ketogenic diet will really help you to lose weight in no time.

So, what you have come to learn from this book is what exactly the ketogenic diet is all about and how you can use it for your own weight loss journey.

You have learned the basics of the ketogenic diet, the benefits of trying it out, how you can use it with intermittent fasting to lose more weight, the foods that are allowed on the ketogenic diet, and even some meal plans to help you get started.

It is important to mention that the more information that you have before starting the ketogenic diet, the more you will be successful with this diet.

Just keep in mind that when you are tired of trying out all the other diet plans that haven't been successful in the past and you want to work with something that will actually work, the ketogenic diet is always a great option for weight loss.

Thanks again for choosing to read my book and I wish you great success with the ketogenic diet.

Health and Fitness
Chief Aim

*Use the following guide for achieving your health and fitness goals.

Step 1

Write down your health and fitness goal(s) and be specific. For example, if you want to lose 10 pounds then write down, "I want to lose 10 pounds."

At the same time, if you want to build muscle, be specific and write down the amount of muscle you want to have. For example, if you want to have 10 pounds of muscle then write down, "I want to have 10 pounds of muscle."

Step 2

Write down the date by which you want to achieve your health and fitness goal(s).

For example, "I will lose 10 pounds by February 2019."

Example two, "I will be able to run 15 miles nonstop by May 2019."

Step 3

Write down what you are willing to sacrifice in order to achieve your health and fitness goals. In addition, write down what are you willing to give back (to the world) in return for achieving your health and fitness goal(s).

For example, "I am willing to give up drinking alcohol, specifically beer for the next 3 months in order to lose 20 pounds of fat. In addition,

I am going to stop watching television after 10:00 PM and I will instead go to sleep early so that I can wake up early and exercise."

"In return for achieving my health and fitness goals, I will serve as a role model inspiring and helping others to also achieve their health and fitness goals by sharing my knowledge, experience and wisdom."

Step 4

Repeat looking and reading over your Health and Fitness Chief Aim every day until you achieve your health and fitness goals. In addition, look and read over your Health and Fitness Chief Aim multiple times a day. Daily repetition is important for achieving any goal.

BODYBUILDING

How to Build the Body of a Greek God

By Epic Rios

Table of Contents

There are no scenarios in which the publisher or the original author of this work can be in any fashion deemed liable for any hardship or damages that may befall them after undertaking information described herein.

Additionally, the information found on the following pages is intended for informational purposes only and should thus be considered, universal.

As befitting its nature, the information presented is without assurance regarding its continued validity or interim quality.

Trademarks that mentioned are done without written consent and can in no way be considered an endorsement from the trademark holder.

Introduction

Congratulations on purchasing your personal copy of *Bodybuilding: How to Build the Body of a Greek God.*

Thank you for doing so.

These days, bodybuilding information is everywhere.

Building muscular big bodies seems to be the norm, but is that really what you are looking for? And at what cost are you willing to build a big body?

This book looks at the classic Greek God physique, one that is strong and capable of achieving great things.

With big, clunky bodies becoming the norm for good physiques these days, it is important to have an alternative for people that don't want a big, overly muscular body.

It is important to state that the ancient Greek body is one that was built on hard work and military training.

In addition, the ancient Greeks did not focus on putting in long hours of weight training at the gym every day.

Instead, the ancient Greeks were hardworking warriors and farmers and their bodies reflected that functionality.

The following chapters will discuss how to create a modern-day workout with focus on the old Greek ways of bodybuilding in order to build a healthy, strong body that is more than just a showpiece.

This book will also discuss specific workouts and nutrition plans that will help you achieve your ideal body.

By reading this book, you will discover how important maintaining an overall healthy lifestyle is in creating an ideal Greek body.

In addition, you will also realize how your mental, physical and overall quality of life will greatly improve as a result of developing and maintaining your new physique.

It is important to state that there are plenty of books on bodybuilding on the market, but none are quite like this.

Thanks again for choosing to purchase this book. Also, every effort was made to ensure this book provides you with as much useful information as possible. Please enjoy!

Chapter 1: Greek Bodies in Art - Drawings and Statues

In order to truly understand what you are striving for with building a Greek physique, it is important to understand the history behind the ideal Greek body, as it is a rich and vibrant one.

First off, the Greek empire existed from 800 BC to 146 BC, about three thousand years ago.

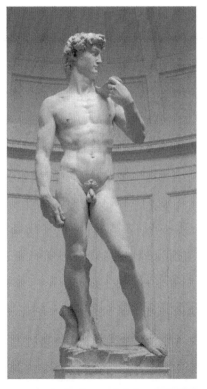

The David, by Michelangelo

Even though it was so long ago, ancient Greek culture is still influencing civilizations around the world, including the modern-day health and fitness culture.

A major theme in Greek art throughout the centuries has been to maintain good order and form.

The goal with any piece of art is to draw the eye and keep it by presenting something that makes sense to the eye and to the brain.

By using subjects that have perfect proportions, the human eye will constantly be drawn to looking at a figure, statue or piece of art.

These concepts of subjects that have perfect proportions have been reflected in the work of well to do modern artists

When it comes to art and statues, the main focus for the ancient Greeks was to create a human form that was IDEAL and PLEASING to the human eye.

According to the ancient Greeks, the Greek body was considered an ideal standard to the ancient Greeks for a number of reasons.

One reason was that the ancient Greeks wanted to have the reputation of being a strong and conquering society portrayed by an ideal Greek body.

Although modern day Greece is very different today than what it used to be, the ancient Greek empire reached all the way to what is now considered the Middle East.

The ancient Greek citizens were considered some of the most fearsome warriors of their time and war was constantly glorified.

The ancient Greeks were very proud of their society and they expressed it through their art by creating Greek Gods with ideal eye-catching proportions.

The strong and pioneering Greek soldiers' body became a model as the ideal Greek.

What is interesting and often forgotten in modern society is that the ancient Greeks manufactured these ideal images in the likeness of Gods in which they have never actually met.

Just like in all religions, the idea of God is just that, an idea.

Although Gods are just figures in a person's imagination, the human mind simply creates an image that it finds appealing and this is something the ancient Greeks were very good at.

The ancient Greeks were very good at developing these ideal Gods that reflected their warrior like society and they were very proud of these ideal Gods.

Although the ancient Greeks creation of Gods and superhuman figures were not born out of reality but out of imagination, the Greeks believed it was their DUTY to uphold and live up to these imaginary images.

These days you will see superhuman figures created by artists using Photoshop that are not a true reflection of modern day society.

Just like the ancient Greeks, modern day society tries to live up to these ideal Photoshop images and people unsuccessfully fail to achieve the ideal body image they want to achieve because these ideal body images are not real.

Simply, many people dream of having a perfect body with perfect form but in nature and in reality, a perfect body doesn't exist.

Even people that have plastic surgery still do not have a perfect body because there will always be a flaw and an imperfection that can be pointed out and recognized.

It is important to state that an important event that made the ancient Greeks very popular was the creation of the Olympics.

When the ancient Greeks established the Olympics, they created games where they could display the strength and stamina of their people.

In addition, the Greeks believed that participating and succeeding at these Olympic games was an important time to display their more than ideal physiques.

While the focus was on winning at the Olympic games, it was a great opportunity for the ancient Greeks to display the beauty and power of their ideal bodies.

The first Olympics was held in honor of Zeus, the most respected of all the Greek Gods.

Interestingly, nudity was common at the Olympic games because the ancient Greeks believed that the human body was something of beauty and should be worshipped.

As a result, the ancient Greeks thought it would be a great idea for participants to display their nude artistic looking physiques during the Olympic games.

The belief system of ancient Greece also brought rise to the idealistic body.

In Greek mythology, a total of fourteen Gods existed, all of which had their own strengths.

Zeus, who was the most powerful of all the Greek Gods, was the God of Thunder and Sky.

There was also Hades, the God of the Underworld, and Apollo, the God of the Sun, among others.

What all the male Greek Gods had in common were their marvelous physiques.

Regardless of their power and personal strength, ancient Greek Gods were portrayed following a natural form that was most physically appealing to the human eye.

Ancient Greek art always depicted the Greeks Gods as perfect creatures, who existed in a form that was in great proportion.

Even today you can see paintings and sculptures that display well-proportioned athletic Greek bodies.

Some of the most famous artworks and sculptures were created during the classical period of Greece, between 500 and 300 B.C.

This period influenced the Roman Empire and had the most lasting impression through art and civilization surviving worldwide in modern times.

The classical period of Greece was also a time in which Greek artists did their best work to recreate the ideal human form thought to be a direct liking to the bodies of Greeks Gods.

During the classical period of Greece, the proper ratios of the human body were extensively studied.

The ancient Greeks were so obsessed with the ideal human form that they were one of the first civilizations to quantify proper ratios of waist to height, waist and shoulder width and other body proportions.

These important body ratios will be discussed in more detail in the next chapter.

Famous works of art like Discobolus, a statue of a Greek athlete throwing a discus, is a very iconic statue that shows a strong and powerful Greek body in action.

This sculpture shows the athletes agility and the body's range of motion as well as the development of muscle and brute strength required to be an ideal figure for the ancient Greeks.

It is important to remember that the Olympics originated in ancient Greece and the Greek athletes were the best of the best.

The ancient Greeks athletic bodies were hard and strong and the athletes were able to participate in all the games, including wresting, boxing and running events.

Another popular ancient Greek sculpture is "The David," created by Michelangelo during the Renaissance period.

This popular ancient Greek sculpture is a work of art that cannot be compared to any other.

"The David" depicts a young man of stellar form simply standing there, at about seventeen feet tall.

With a modest smile and oblivious attitude, this young man is simply in all his glory; a Greek man.

The musculature and details of "The David" show a man in his true, perfect form.

Speaking of Michelangelo, he was also responsible for creating beautiful works of art in the Sistine Chapel in Vatican City.

Michelangelo's painting on the ceiling of the Sistine Chapel in Vatican City called, "The Creation of Adam" is one of the most famous pieces of art ever created.

This famous piece of art shows an iconic image of when God first created Adam, the first human.

It shows the hands of God and Adam reaching out to each other to touch each other's hands.

It is important to state that the bodies of both Adam and God are shown in ideal proportions, typical of ancient Greek art.

In addition, you can clearly see the purity of both figures because they have been painted in a way that depicts flawless bodies; something to be attained.

Interestingly, the bodies of ancient Greek women and goddesses are idealized in a much different way than we see in modern times.

Modern day's standard of beauty says that women should be very thin yet display a bit of muscularity.

Looking at ancient Greek art, we cannot compare these modern standards to the influences from ancient Greece.

In fact, ancient Greek women were idolized for being slender but not "sickly" thin like modern day female "models."

Ancient Greek women were in proper proportion with their waists. They were slender but their hips were large and showed the ability to bear children.

Ancient Greek women were known to be healthy and it was very important in ancient Greece for women to have a healthy figure for bearing children.

In addition, there were no chiseled female chins or emphasis on rock hard abs like modern day female bodybuilders or women CrossFit warriors.

Instead, ancient Greece was a more lenient time for women, as womens primary role was to bear children and serve as a caregiver.

Similarly, the standard for the male physique, since ancient Greek times, has also changed as well.

For example, there was a major shift in the late twentieth century that morphed the ideal ancient Greek male figure into that of a superhero.

So late twentieth century male fitness figures would begin to have muscles that were required to be big and overdeveloped regardless of being functional.

In addition, late twentieth century male fitness figures would be bulky and their upper bodies were much larger than their lower bodies.

Think of modern day bodybuilders and men who use steroids to gain mass, yet lack function and athleticism.

Modern day overly developed muscular bodies are so far against the ideal, functional warrior body of the ancient Greek.

These days, we have traded function and athleticism for "gym and beach muscles," specifically the chest and arm muscles.

In addition, many modern-day bodybuilders can bench press 300 pounds but they don't have the functionality to carry a suitcase up the stairs or lack the conditioning to run 1 mile at an easy pace.

For the ancient Greeks, they took great pride in having the ability to use their ideal bodies to fight in wars, maintain their homes and provide food for their families.

It is important to state that the ancient Greeks did not have any modern-day tools or equipment to do any heavy lifting of objects or structures.

Instead, the ancient Greeks simply used brute strength and a strong willingness to move, function, complete any task and survive on a daily basis.

Chapter 2: Proportions of Greek Gods

Ancient Greeks took their physiques very seriously.

For the ancient Greeks, it was considered a sign of strength, power and strong character to maintain a certain physique.

This was modeled after the perfection of Greek Gods, who were considered immortal and strong by the ancient Greeks.

The ancient Greeks even went as far as to consider specific measurements of the human body to be desirable.

Much like bodybuilders today, the ancient Greeks were obsessed with obtaining a perfect body.

However, unlike modern day bodybuilders, the perfect Greek body was one that was functional, athletic and strong.

It is important to state that ancient Greece was often in war and it needed healthy, strong warriors to maintain their armies and fight their enemies.

As a result, the ancient Greeks trained as fearless warriors and it was deemed necessary to have a strong, functional body to even have a fighting chance against their enemies.

Ancient Greek men trained to be powerful, agile and fast in order to defeat their enemies.

Fearless Greek warriors were naturally lean, carrying very little body fat. They also had strong upper bodies but did not have overly developed chest and arm muscles like current day bodybuilders.

It was important for ancient Greek warriors to have great stamina in order to run and be able to travel on foot to new battle fields to fight against their enemies.

Stamina was a huge part of training for ancient Greek warriors.

Being able to run long distances to a battle field without getting tired and then upon arrival be ready to fight with NO REST was an absolute must for an ancient Greek warrior.

Those Greek warriors who did not have the stamina to keep up with the rest of the Greek warriors would be left behind and would be the first to die in battle.

For the ancient Greek warriors, they simply trained to survive and not just to look good naked.

These days, there are fewer opportunities to fight in battle. In addition, modern day armies have available vehicles and planes to move people around as well as sophisticated weaponry to prevent hand to hand combat.

As a result, there is no real reason for any modern day "soldier" to really train as a warrior when sophisticated technology can do all the fighting for them.

It is important to state that ancient Greek warriors were often in face-to-face combat with their enemies, using swords and shields as their weapons.

In addition, the Greek warriors were required to have tremendous strength and stamina in order to use their swords and shields effectively in battle without getting tired.

Even Greek men who were not part of the Greek military and did not fight in battle were considered strong, athletic and ready for battle if needed.

Those Greek men who were not fighting were farmers and workers who spent their days working in the fields, growing crops and responsible for the agriculture of ancient Greece.

These Greek men working in the fields were tough. They would work long days lifting crops and items over their heads while pulling on their livestock at the same time.

These Greek famers rarely were in situations in which they would need to bench press weights or perform barbell curls.

Instead, these Greek farmers had functional strength, the kind that is required for every day survival and that is required for getting real work done.

It is important to state that the ideal measurements of a strong working Greek man were as follows: for the bicep it was **16.4 inches in diameter**.

As compared to a modern bodybuilder, a strong working Greek man's bicep is considered small.

In addition, during the ancient Greek era, the ideal neck for a Greek man was **16.8 inches in diameter,** the ideal chest was **45.5-inches in diameter** and the ideal forearms were **13.2 inches in diameter.**

These ideal measurements seem like very specific body ratios to aim for but if you were a Greek man, reaching these goals was a matter of day to day survival and living.

As for the lower body ideal measurements for a Greek man, it is first important to state that the ancient Greeks had naturally strong and muscular legs.

In addition, ancient Greek men were required to be able to run long distances, be agile enough to evade enemies and strong enough to work as farmers and perform daily chores.

As a result, a Greek man was required to have legs that were functional and not overly muscular or bulky in order to remain functional for day to day living.

The lower body ideal measurements for a Greek man are as follows:

A perfect thigh was **24.1 inches in diameter** and the calf muscle was **15.5 inches in diameter.**

Now that you know a little about the ancient Greeks upper and lower body ideal measurements, let us now focus on the abdomen.

The ancient Greeks were known to have a very strong core.

As you may or may not know, the abdomen and back are the muscles at the center of every physical movement.

The abdomen allows for the arms and legs to swing in a controlled manner.

The ancient Greeks were known to have slim athletic bodies that were not overly built. In addition, their waists were in direction proportion to the rest of their bodies.

An ideal perfect waist for a Greek man was **31.9 inches in diameter** and an ideal perfect hip ratio was **38.7 inches in diameter**.

Hearing about the ancient Greeks perfect body measurements may seem like a bit of a turn-off.

In addition, you may ask yourself, "How on earth is an everyday person able to achieve such ideal body standards?"

Truthfully, it is very difficult to achieve the ancient Greeks ideal body standards because everyone's body type and bone structure is different.

However, once you know your body type, you can then work on developing a near perfect body like the ancient Greeks.

If you don't know what your body type is consider that there are three body types that most people are considered to fit into.

The three body types are:
1. Ectomorph
2. Mesomorph and
3. Endomorph

An **Ectomorph** is a person that is naturally thin and has a very thin bone structure.

In addition, an Ectomorph may have a hard time gaining weight and as a result a person with this body type remains naturally thin.

A **Mesomorph** is a person that has more of a "desired" body type because this person is neither thin nor big but instead this body type fits perfectly between an **Ectomorph** and an **Endomorph**.

An **Endomorph** is a person that has more of a "round shape" body type. In addition, the bone structure of this body type tends to be bigger and wider than the other body types.

Once you figure out which body type you may have, you can then work on creating a physique like the ancient Greeks according to your body type.

As you learn about the ancient Greeks ideal body measurements and their obsession with the human body, it is important to state that you should not get discouraged with achieving your health and fitness goals.

In all honestly, it will be very difficult to attain and maintain a body like the ancient Greeks believed a human body should look like so don't focus too much on these ideal body measurements.

Instead, consider the **Golden Ratio**, a term and a number that is much simpler to understand.

The Golden Ratio is a mathematical figure that was used during ancient Greece that many artists often believed expressed an ideal body displaying both beauty and balance.

As a result, the Golden Ratio was used to portray balance and beauty in many paintings and sculptures during the Renaissance period.

It is even said that Da Vinci himself used the Golden Ratio for defining all the proportions and dimensions for his paintings.

As you can see, the ideal body proportions of ancient Greek statues are a reflection of the Golden Ratio.

So rather than focusing on obtaining ideal body measurements according to the ancient Greeks, it is a lot more important to look at the overall proportions of your very own measurements.

However, modern research shows that when it comes to human attraction, men who fit a certain "ideal body ratio" are considered scientifically more attractive to women.

For example, the ancient Greek male physique was known to have broad shoulders with a narrow waist and hips that produced a "V-shaped" look.

And even in modern times, research shows that men that display a "V-shaped" look are considered more attractive by women.

What can also be said about the ideal body measurements of the ancient Greeks was that they believed it was very important for the neck, arms and calves to all have the same measurements in order to contribute to the ideal Greek body type.

The ancient Greeks believed so strongly that their perception of ideal body measurements were very attractive and pleasing to the human eye and so that is why they regarded them so highly.

It can be said that the same way the Golden Ratio was used to expressed an ideal body during ancient Greek times, the human face also follows a similar ratio.

For example, research shows that ideal facial features should be symmetrical and aligned in a way that follows a natural order.

In addition, faces that are symmetrical and aligned well are considered the most attractive.

To develop a body that is ideal to your proportions consider that your waist circumference should be 40-50% of your height.

So, if you are six feet tall, or 72 inches tall, your ideal waist size is between 28 and 36 inches.

Knowing your ideal waist size can help you determine your ideal shoulder size as well.

If you exercise and you truly want to make sure your overall body is well proportioned without being overly muscular or bulky, simply consider your lower body to be well proportioned to your upper body.

So, you don't want to have an overdeveloped upper body and an underdeveloped lower body.

Instead, you want to train to make sure your upper and lower body are well proportioned to each other.

You also want to consider that your calves should measure about the same as your biceps and your thighs should be strong yet slender.

Sometimes people are naturally born with big calves and legs but this does not mean that your arms and biceps should be equally as big.

Naturally, the human body can only get so muscular without steroids.

So, if you are looking to develop a naturally looking, well-proportioned body like the ancient Greeks, then aim for developing a body that is more "athletic" looking vs a bodybuilder's physique.

To put things in perspective, the ideal Greek body was described as one with broad shoulders, strong and without overly developed arms.

In addition, the chest was required to be strong, tapering down to a slim, yet muscular core. And the legs of an ideal Greek physique were required to be muscular but lean.

The ideal Greek physique was meant to be functional and ready for war and not meant to be shown off for vanity.

Nowadays, many men enjoy wearing tighter clothing that helps them show off their physiques and that is simply because they are trying to attract women or impress people.

Keep in mind that in clothes, a modern day Greek body looks slender but toned. In addition, there should be no bulging muscles trying to escape your t-shirt.

Remember that we all have certain features about ourselves that we cannot change.

Things dictated by our genetics like the shape of our faces or the proportions of our bone structures cannot be changed unless you are considering plastic surgery.

What you can do is use good nutrition and total body workouts to develop toned muscles and reduce your body fat percentage.

If you want to develop a body like the ancient Greeks then use the ideal ancient Greek physique as a benchmark in order to guide yourself with the proper nutrition and training that is required.

It is important to state that obtaining a near perfect body like the ancient Greeks may be very difficult to achieve.

Instead, focus on improving your health and fitness levels and enjoy yourself along the process.

Chapter 3: How Hollywood Portrays Greek Gods

Although a lot of things have changed since ancient Greece, our physical bodies and body types have not.

In addition, it is still very possible to achieve a body like the ancient Greeks but it does require a lot of hard work and commitment.

Just take Hollywood actors for example.

There are many Hollywood actors that have been able to achieve a body similar to the ancient Greeks and this has been clearly portrayed in movies.

Hollywood actors have even gone so far as to develop bodies that are strong and functional similar to the ancient Greeks.

Remember, the ancient Greeks were required to have a strong body yet its primary purpose was to be "functional."

If you look at famous Hollywood actor Brad Pitt, he was able to transform himself into a Godlike warrior known as "Achilles" in the movie "Troy."

In the movie "Troy," "Achilles" is known for being a fierce warrior that displayed great strength and agility.

If you analyze Brad Pitt's physique in the movie "Troy," you do not see him with bulging bodybuilder type of muscles.

Instead, his muscles are toned and he is very athletic displaying tremendous speed, power and agility.

In addition, Brad Pitt's midsection is long and lean with strong, well-chiseled arms and legs.

Although the physiques of Hollywood actors may not always seem to be realistic, what can be said is that with proper nutrition, training and exercise, an average looking person can most certainly transform themselves to look like a modern day athletic Greek warrior.

Another Brad Pitt movie that has become a "classic" among men as a result of his godlike body is the 1999 movie "Fight Club."

In the movie "Fight Club," Brad Pitt plays the role of "Tyler Durden," the founding member of an underground fight club where members of the group fight each other bare knuckled and without rules.

Although the role that Brad Pitt plays in the movie "Fight Club" is very different then the role he played in the movie "Troy," he is still able to display an amazing godlike physique in the movie "Fight Club."

For example, in the movie "Fight Club," Brad Pitt has a very long but lean, athletic body almost displaying more of a "boxer's" physique.

In addition, Brad Pitt appears to be very "cut" and able to display very defined 6-pack abs in the movie "Fight Club."

"Tyler Durden," as Brad Pitt is referred to in the movie "Fight Club" is meant to look scrappy, squirrely and a little bit crazy.

In addition, Brad Pitt's face is chiseled as a result of having very little body fat and his muscles are well defined.

Overall, Brad Pitt's body in the movie "Fight Club" is designed to show that it is meant for fighting and destroying others.

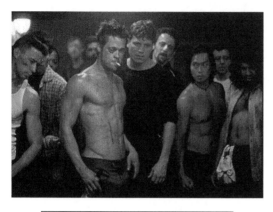

There are many fascinating movies that show ancient warriors with godlike physiques like the movie "Troy" and the very popular "300" which is about the famous 300 Spartans.

Brad Pitt, Fight Club

However, in the past few years, Superhero movies have become quite popular with many people as a result of the action in the movies and the muscular physiques of the Superheroes.

It is important to state that there is a great distinction between the ancient Greek God body and the Superhero body.

While the ancient Greek God body and the Superhero body are both strong and muscular, the Superhero body is very similar to the body of a modern-day bodybuilder.

It is important to state that the art of Bodybuilding slowly became more and more popular in the 1940s.

In addition, there was a massive push by the bodybuilders to display just how big their muscles can get.

Bodybuilders, since the 1940's have focused on developing extremely large upper bodies while maintaining very tiny waists.

In addition, the idea of having proper Greek proportions was totally disregarded and forgotten by bodybuilders.

Bodybuilders also focused on pure aesthetics disregarding developing a "functional" physique which was the result of hard work by the ancient Greeks.

Bodybuilding competitions also quickly took off in the 1940's with top contenders having very large, sometimes steroid induced chest and bicep muscles with tiny, almost womanlike waists.

Bodybuilders later began to use tanning products and baby oil during bodybuilding competitions for the purpose of enhancing muscle definition.

Back in the days of the ancient Greeks, there was no need for using tanning products and baby oil for the purpose of displaying a well-defined physique.

Instead, the ancient Greeks developed an aesthetically warriorlike physique as a result of every day hard work and survival.

While a bit exaggerated, the Superhero body, which can be currently seen in several movies, has adopted more of a bodybuilder's physique then the ancient Greek God warrior physique.

This is because every year we see more and more people pushing their bodies to get bigger and bigger with the help of steroids and performance enhancing drugs.

As a result, having a big bulky body has become the norm in the fitness and entertainment industries including Hollywood's portrayal of Superheroes and their bodybuilder type physiques in movies like Captain America and Thor.

These days, Marvel Comics and other comic book giants have made movies of just about every Superhero out there.

Popular Superheroes like Superman and Thor are displayed on covers of DVDs all over the world. Their upper bodies are large and in charge, almost carrying too much muscle to be of any real help.

Chris Hemsworth, the actor that plays Thor in the most recent Avengers series has a typical modern day overly muscular superhero build.

While his muscles and physique are something to be admired, the look of his body is very different from the ideal ancient Greek warrior physique.

Even today, cartoon depictions of superheroes are even more exaggerated than ever.

Take a look at the character "Metroman" in the Dreamworks movie "Megamind."

"Metroman" has a huge upper body and a very small waist and very thin legs.

Yes, "Metroman" is just a cartoon character but this overly muscular cartoon Superhero reinforces the idea that having a large upper body is the new standard of strength when it comes to Superheroes even if it is just a cartoon.

Chapter 4: Build Muscle Like a Greek God

Getting the body of a Greek God may actually be easier and more productive than you think.

Remember that ancient Greek ideal bodies were that of functional human beings. So, this means that the ancient Greeks did NOT have ideal bodies for the mere purpose of showing off their muscles.

Instead, the ancient Greeks were proud of their physiques as a result of training hard every day as warriors ready for battle.

In addition, the ancient Greeks also worked very hard in the fields growing crops to feed their families.

As you can see, the ancient Greeks were able to build muscle by doing physical labor and not by counting endless repetitions in a weight room.

Now in order to develop a workout routine that will help you develop a physique like the ancient Greek warriors, it is important to first consider exactly what the ancient Greeks did to develop their physiques.

In addition, it is also important to consider how to go about naturally transforming your body whether at home or at a gym.

There are currently many fitness companies and gyms that exist that purposely (or not) design exercise routines that build strength through functional exercise.

Perhaps the most popular right now is CrossFit.

Another popular fitness organization that helps fitness enthusiasts to build strength through functional exercise is the Ultimate Fighting Championship or (UFC).

Although you may not have the desire to be a UFC fighter, training in mixed martial arts is an excellent way for developing a warriorlike physique similar to the ancient Greeks.

So, in order to develop a body like the ancient Greeks you have to consider what kinds of functional exercises are required to develop a warriorlike physique.

Some good functional exercises are bodyweight exercises such as:
1. Pull-ups
2. Parallel bar dips
3. Pushups
4. Bodyweight squats
5. Jumping squats
6. Lunges
7. Jumping lunges

Some good functional exercises using fitness equipment can be:
1. Medicine ball exercises such as medicine ball throws
2. Kettlebell exercises such as kettlebell walks or "farmer walks"
3. Dumbbell exercises such as dumbbell squats to shoulder press
4. Jump rope exercises such as explosive jump roping with "double unders" and "criss-crosses"

Remember that the ancient Greeks did not rely on heavy equipment for getting in shape. Instead, they would run, wrestle, box and use brute strength to move large objects.

However, modern day gyms provide a wide variety of training equipment for getting in shape and it is just a matter of learning how to use the equipment for developing a functional body.

It is important to state that the ancient Greeks placed great emphasis on cardio and having the conditioning to run far distances without getting tired was very important to the ancient Greeks.

Some great cardio exercises that would greatly improve your conditioning are:
1. Circuit training using dumbbells, medicine balls, bodyweight exercises or machines
2. Stair running or Running Sprints
3. Using an Indoor Rowing Machine
4. Jump Roping or Skipping Rope
5. Mixed Martials Arts – Specifically Boxing, Muay Thai or Wrestling
6. Plyometric Exercises like jumping squats and burpees

As you can see, a combination of functional strength training exercises combined with effective cardio exercises would make you very athletic and functional.

In addition, a combination of both strength training and cardio type of exercises will most definitely help you develop a physique like the ancient Greeks.

While we will discuss cardio in more detail in the next chapter, just remember that it needs to be integrated into your training routines for developing a lean, functional physique.

That being said, a fitness trend that has become very popular in the fitness world is High Intensity Interval Training or HIIT for short.

High Intensity Interval Training, or HIIT combines small bursts of intense cardio activity usually between 20-90 seconds followed by some rest.

What makes High Intensity Interval Training so popular with many fitness enthusiasts is that it burns fat and can even build muscle in a short amount of time.

You can even do bodyweight exercises and use kettlebells, medicine balls or dumbbells for getting a good high intensity interval training workout.

When it comes to developing a modern-day warrior body like the ancient Greeks it is important to consider what muscles to exercise in order to get the best and fastest results.

Something to keep in mind is that the three largest muscles of the human body are the **legs, back and chest muscles.**

So, when you exercise you want to make sure you focus on exercising these three large muscle groups.

To develop a well-rounded functional body like the ancient Greeks, it is important to consider doing **total body strength training exercises** that work the three largest muscles in the body.

In addition, making effective cardio workouts part of your fitness training will greatly improve your results of achieving a well-rounded functional body like the ancient Greeks.

It is important to state that traditional bodybuilding focuses too much on getting big muscles and displaying overly developed bodies that serve no real-world purpose.

As a result, if you truly want to develop a physique like the ancient Greeks then it is important to train your body to be a lean, functional athletic machine that is ready for anything.

Here are some sample workouts routines that you can use to get you started with your fitness training:

Bodyweight Routine I
1. Chin-ups (5-8 repetitions)
2. Pushups (8-10 repetitions)
3. Lunges (12-15 repetitions)

Rest for 30-40 seconds and repeat for 5 sets
Perform each exercise one after the other with no rest

Circuit Training Routine II
1. Dumbbell Goblet squats (10-15 repetitions)
2. Dumbbell rows (8-12 repetitions)
3. Dumbbell bench press (8-12 repetitions)
4. Dumbbell lunges (10-15 repetitions)
5. 30 second plank (abs) exercise

Rest for 30-40 seconds and repeat for 5 sets
* Perform each exercise one after the other with no rest*

Strength and Plyometric Training Routine III
1. "farmer walks" using dumbbells or kettlebells
2. Jump rope for 1 minute

Rest for 30-40 seconds and repeat for 5 sets

As you can see from the three sample training routines, these methods of training are very different compared to bodybuilding routines.

While the ancient Greeks had their methods of training for getting fit, it is important for you to develop your own methods, routines and training for developing your own physique.

Remember, the key to a Greek body is training that requires moderate weight for strength training for the purpose of building firm and functional muscles.

Keep in mind that making the goal to lift as much weight as humanly possible will get you more of a superhero type of body instead of a Greek warrior body.

Always keep the goal in mind to build functional strength without overdoing it.

The good news is, you don't need to spend countless hours at the gym to get a great body.

Instead, you just need to train in a manner that keeps you lean and fit.

In addition, seek to always be "evolving" with your training in order to remain motivated with achieving your health and fitness goals.

Another thing to consider is that weight training in the gym no longer means you have to be doing the so called, "best exercises" for getting fit.

Instead, think about the fitness goals you want to achieve. Next, develop a plan to achieve your fitness goals. Finally, take action for achieving your fitness goals.

So, if your fitness goals are to develop a body like a Greek warrior, then train in a functional manner that will produce those results.

In addition, don't fall into the trap of having to do certain or specific exercises for getting in shape.

Instead, experiment with a variety of exercises, fitness routines and training equipment for getting the best results when it comes to achieving your fitness goals.

Consider that the ancient Greeks did not perform exercises like the barbell squat or deadlift because squatting heavy weight and deadlifting did not serve them any purpose in battle or in everyday living.

Simply the bodies of the ancient Greeks were not built for squatting or deadlifting hundreds of pounds, repetition after repetition because for them it was unnecessary to do so.

Just looking at an ideal Greek figure, we can tell that the ancient Greeks were not bench pressing excessive weight, as their chests were defined but not huge like modern day bodybuilders.

While using weight machines and free weights can mimic functional exercise, it can only go so far.

This is why interval training and doing activities that combine muscle training with real life situations is so important.

Remember, interval training is a method of doing a combination of high intense exercise followed by low intense exercise.

For example, running sprints for 50 yards giving 100% effort followed by very light jogging giving 50% effort would be considered interval training.

As you can see by this example of interval training, this type of training would have been beneficial to the ancient Greeks especially during wartime.

Although in the beginning, there were no available gyms in ancient Greece for Greek warriors to train, Greek warriors simply trained outside in public view.

Eventually, training in public view led to establishments for training and learning which later became known as "Gymnasiums."

The ancient Greeks believed the human body was such a beautiful art form that they would even go so far as to exercise naked at Gymnasiums.

Something to keep in mind is that whenever ancient Greek warriors did train, they never counted repetitions.

Instead, the ancient Greeks trained to simply improve their fitness levels as well as for preparing themselves for warfare.

It is important to state that Greek warriors would practice fighting, boxing, wrestling and they practiced training to fight using their powerful swords.

Today, we can recreate some of this type of training with mixed martial arts training.

When it comes to developing a body like an ancient Greek warrior, consider focusing your time on taking classes that combine lots of disciplines and training that the ancient Greeks would likely be doing.

For example, you can seek to improve your flexibility by learning Yoga. You can also seek to improve your breathing and your ability to relax and concentrate by practicing meditation.

You can even expand on your athletic pursuits by learning new fitness skills like advanced calisthenics or learning how to swim like a pro.

The most important thing you must do for developing a body like an ancient Greek warrior is to simply take action.

In addition, develop a strong willingness for achieving your Greek warrior physique and don't make excuses.

What is great about this very moment is that we are living in a time where we have access to all kinds of fitness training, state of the art gyms and equipment.

In addition, there is an abundance of available information on nutrition, dieting and overall health.

Therefore, it is a lot easier NOW to build a functional physique than it was when the ancient Greeks did it.

It is important to state that there is no one specific way for developing a body like the ancient Greeks.

To build a functional and well-proportioned body like the ancient Greeks consider the following steps:

1) **Develop a plan for getting fit.** This includes the types of exercises you will do, the type of equipment you will use, how often you will exercise and for how long you will exercise for.

2) **Focus on your nutrition.** Nutrition is extremely important for developing a lean, functional physique like the ancient Greeks.

   Consider what foods you will be required to eat for getting lean and fit. We will discuss nutrition later in the following chapters.

3) **Make a commitment.** Make a commitment to yourself for taking the necessary action and following through with achieving the body you want to have.

   In addition, consider how you will transform your body and look in 3 months, 6 months, 9 months and in 1 year.

Following these steps will most definitely help you to build a functional and well-proportioned body like the ancient Greeks

As stated before, there is no one specific way for developing a body like the ancient Greeks.

Instead it is a matter of experimenting with different types of exercises, equipment, fitness routines and training.

Many people believe that going to a gym and lifting heavy weights is the only way for developing a lean, functional physique but this is not true.

Instead, consider that you can exercise at home using bodyweight exercises. You can also exercise outside running sprints.

You can even do a combination of running sprints and then perform bodyweight exercises like pushups while you rest.

It is important to use your creative mind for getting lean and developing a functional body.

When you use your creative mind for getting lean and fit, you develop a sense of curiosity for seeing what is possible.

In addition, you learn more about what you can achieve both physically and mentally when you use your creative mind for getting fit.

You also keep yourself motivated along your journey for developing and achieving the type of body you want to have.

Below are 3 very important areas you want to focus on when developing your Greek warrior physique:

1) **Strength** – Strength is important for having a strong body. However, lifting extremely heavy weight is not required for developing a lean, functional physique.

   Instead, simply focus on doing what is challenging for you and always keep safety in mind.

2) **Conditioning -** Conditioning is important because it allows you to develop endurance so that you will not get tired so easily and so that you can push through your workouts.

   In addition, it is not enough to simply develop a good-looking body. Instead, developing a functional body, a body that is useful, a body that does not get tired so easily is the goal behind developing a Greek warrior physique.

3) **Flexibility** – Flexibility is important because it prevents your body from getting very stiff and losing its range of motion.

   In addition, you will have more mobility and you will move better as a result of having more flexibility. You will also avoid injuries as a result of developing more flexibility throughout your body.

As you can see, focusing on developing strength, conditioning and flexibility will help you develop the physique of an ancient Greek warrior.

In addition, you will become lean, functional and athletic as a result of focusing on strength, conditioning and flexibly.

To give you an example of how one particular Greek God was able to develop his lean, functional body, let's look at Poseidon, the God of the Sea, Horses, Storms and Earthquakes.

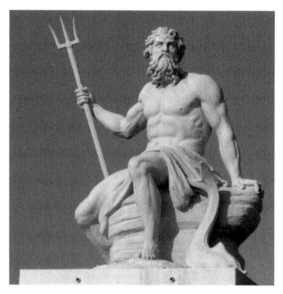

Poseidon, God of the Sea

Poseidon, was most notably known as God of the Sea and protector of all waters because of his excellent swimming abilities.

Poseidon had the ability to stay underwater for long periods of time.

In addition, Poseidon was also known as an "Olympian God" that participated in the ancient Greek Olympic Games.

Poseidon was strong, athletic and resembled Zeus, the God of Sky and Thunder.

Now some people may be thinking, "How can swimming help me develop the body of a Greek warrior?"

In addition, some people may consider swimming to be more of a cardio type of exercise instead of a strength training exercise. However, this is simply not true.

Swimming is a unique total body workout that can help you develop speed, balance, agility, coordination, strength and improve your overall athleticism.

Now you may be asking, "But what if I don't know how to swim?"

Consider that in the past ten years, more and more athletic coaches have been making swimming pool workouts part of their athletes training and recovery programs.

For example, aside from using a swimming pool to simply swim sprints and perform various swim strokes, you can actually run in a swimming pool both in the shallow and deep end.

You can also perform plyometric exercises in a swimming pool such as jumping squats, jumping lunges and tuck squats.

You can also do resistance training exercises in a swimming pool using your own bodyweight, specialized dumbbells and other training equipment.

As stated before, there is NO one specific way for developing a physique like the ancient Greeks.

Therefore, it is important to keep an open mind, experiment with various exercises, training and workouts and stay committed to achieving your health and fitness goals.

Chapter 5: Cutting Fat with Cardio

Getting lean, fit and developing a functional body is what is required for developing a physique like the ancient Greeks.

However, for many people getting extremely lean is very difficult to do especially in modern times because of easy access to all kinds of unhealthy foods.

Keep in mind that when you exercise you will develop some muscle. But unless you focus on developing a lean body, then that muscle will remain hiding behind a layer of body fat.

We already talked a lot about how muscle tone is essential for having an ideal Greek body. However, it is important to state that body fat plays a major role on how your body looks.

As mentioned in a previous chapter, the ancient Greeks were fanatics about having perfect body proportions.

Now keep this in mind…adding fat to any area of the body even a lit bit of fat will change your body ratios.

It is understandable that every person carries weight a little differently, leading to a couple of extra inches here and there.

For example, men that overeat tend to gain weight around their stomach and chest areas and women that overeat tend to gain weight around their hips and thighs.

In addition, we previously talked a little bit about the **3 body types** that people fit into which are **Ectomorph, Mesomorph and Endomorph**.

Ectomorphs are known as "hard gainers," because they can eat a lot of food but they have a hard time putting on weight.

Now, if you look at an **Endomorph**, it is very easy for them to gain weight so they have to be more cautious about what they eat.

It is important to state that your DIET is more important than exercise!

Many people believe that they can eat whatever they want and then easily burn those calories with exercise and this is simply not true.

Stop and think about how many calories are in some of your favorite foods.

Here are some examples of calories in different foods:

1. **A Big Mac has around 490 calories.** To burn those 490 calories, you will have to do 1 hour of intense strength training exercise or 42 minutes of intense cardio exercise.

2. **A pint of beer has 245 calories.** To burn off those 245 calories you would have to do 30 minutes of strength training exercise or 21 minutes of intense cardio exercise.

3. **2 slices of cheese pizza have around 600 calories.** To burn those 600 calories, you would have to swim 1 full hour to burn off those 2 slices of cheese pizza.

4. **4 small chocolate chip cookies have around 213 calories.** To burn those 213 calories, you would have to run 23 minutes on a treadmill.

5. **A small bag of potato chips has around 262 calories.** Now to burn those 262 calories you would have to walk 1 hour and 13 minutes.

6. **A small cup of vanilla and chocolate ice-cream has an estimated 540 calories.** Now to burn those 540 calories you would have to ride a bicycle for 1 hour and 22 minutes.

These examples of foods and their calorie amounts do not take into consideration all the other foods you eat on a daily basis as well as the amount of exercise you will need to do in order to burn those calories.

In order to truly obtain the physique of an ancient Greek warrior it is important to be mindful of your nutrition and eating habits. We will talk more about nutrition in the following chapters.

But for the moment, consider that although strength training exercises like bodyweight exercises will help you to build muscle it is also important to make cardio exercises part of your fitness training.

Making cardio exercises part of your fitness training is great for your body and health because cardio will help you to build stamina and reduce some of your bodyfat.

Although achieving a lean fit body is definitely a goal to aim at, it is important to state that having some body fat is actually good for your body and health.

For example, having small amounts of bodyfat is necessary for protecting your vital organs.

In addition, body fat provides your body with nutrients, gives you energy, helps with sport performance along with many other benefits.

Although you cannot completely eliminate bodyfat, you can definitely keep your bodyfat levels in check.

Keep this in mind…if you want to be lean, fit and functional, aim to have a low but healthy amount of bodyfat.

Having a low but healthy amount of bodyfat will give you a well-defined look to your physique.

So, want you want to do is tone and strengthen your entire body. In addition, you want to reduce some of your bodyfat with cardiovascular exercise.

As we have learned from ancient Greek art, the ideal Greek body was toned and lean, not weak and flabby.

It is important to state that the **ideal Greek bodyfat percentage** was about **10% fat** which is a good bodyfat percentage to have because it is low enough for displaying a toned, well-defined athletic body.

In addition, 10% bodyfat is quite a healthy bodyfat percentage to have because it is neither too low, nor too high.

Here is a chart showing bodyfat percentages for both men and women:

Ideal Bodyfat Percentage Chart

Description	Men	Women
Essential bodyfat	2-5% bodyfat (is not safe)	10-13% bodyfat (is not safe)
*Athletes	*6 - 13% bodyfat (is Ideal)	*14 - 20% bodyfat (is Ideal)
Casual Fitness	14-17% bodyfat	21-24% bodyfat
Average Person	18-24% bodyfat	24-31% bodyfat
Obese/Overweight	25% or more bodyfat	32% or more bodyfat

As you can see from the bodyfat percentage chart, having **6-13% bodyfat for men** and **14-20% bodyfat for women** is what you what to aim for when it comes to having an ideal bodyfat percentage.

Although the ideal bodyfat percentages for both men and women may seem difficult achieve it is important to state that it is greatly possible to achieve a low but healthy bodyfat percentage.

It addition, with hard work, good nutrition and making a commitment to get lean and fit, you can definitely achieve the goal of developing the body of an ancient Greek warrior.

As stated before, strength training will tone the body but cardiovascular exercise will "lean out" the body.

There are two types of cardiovascular exercises you want to include as part of your fitness training.

The first type is **aerobic exercise** and the second type is **anaerobic exercise**.

Aerobic exercise is any physical activity that consists of low intensity exercise that lasts for long periods of time.

For example, doing any physical exercise at a low intensity for 10, 20, 30 minutes or more would be considered aerobic exercise.

Some examples of aerobic exercise are running, swimming or cycling at a low intensity.

Now **anaerobic exercise** is intense, fast paced physical activity that is done in a short amount of time.

For example, running or swimming sprints at a full 100% capacity for very short distances are considered anaerobic exercises.

Anaerobic exercise is great for developing strength, speed and power whereas aerobic exercise is good for developing endurance.

Although some people may choose aerobic exercise over anaerobic exercise it is a good idea to do both in order to achieve the best weight loss results.

In addition, doing both aerobic and anaerobic exercise with make you more functional and athletic.

A great benefit of performing both aerobic and anaerobic exercises is that they will strengthen the heart and burn fat at the same time.

In order to get the best result for performing both aerobic and anaerobic exercises, it is a good idea to eat some healthy carbohydrates or "carbs."

Eating healthy carbohydrates will give your body the necessary energy it needs to perform both aerobic and anaerobic exercises effectively.

Although carbohydrates have developed a bad reputation in the past few years, many people seem too mix up the bad carbohydrates with the good carbohydrates.

Here is a short list of some good healthy carbohydrates that you want to eat:

Good Healthy Carbohydrates
1. Sweet Potatoes
2. Legumes, Lentils and Beans
3. Unprocessed Grains like Steel Cut Oats, Brown Rice and Quinoa
4. Fruits and Vegetables

Now that you know what carbohydrates are good for you to eat, lets look at a short list of some bad carbohydrates you want to stay away from:

Bad Unhealthy Carbohydrates
1. White bread
2. Bagels and Muffins
3. French Fries
4. Cakes and cookies
5. Sodas and Juices

As you can see from the list of bad unhealthy carbohydrates you want to stay away from, these are commonly eaten by many people.

What you want to do is try to only eat good healthy carbohydrates because they will give you the necessary energy and vitamins that your body needs for performing at your very best when it comes to cardiovascular exercise and overall exercise.

In addition, you want to remove unhealthy carbohydrates from your diet because they will make you gain weight and negatively affect your athletic performance.

As stated before, eating good healthy carbohydrates will give you the energy you need for performing at your very best when working out.

But something that is important to mention is that eating too many healthy carbohydrates can lead to weight gain especially if you don't use that energy.

So, what you want to do is make sure you only eat enough carbohydrates to fuel your workouts.

It is important to state that eating excess carbohydrates even excess protein can lead to weight gain so it is important to make sure you monitor your food intake.

One eating method that has become popular with many people that live a health and fitness lifestyle is the **Intermittent Fasting lifestyle**.

Living an Intermittent Fasting lifestyle while pursuing your goal of developing the physique of an ancient Greek warrior is a great idea.

You will be able to reduce your bodyfat percentage while developing a functional, athletic body as a result of practicing Intermittent Fasting.

In addition, you can even perform cardiovascular exercise while practicing Intermittent Fasting which will lead to rapid fat loss.

If you don't want to practice Intermittent Fasting but you want to make sure you are still able to burn fat effectively, then consider the Ketogenic Diet as an alternative.

The only downside to the Ketogenic Diet is that because it requires you to eat very few carbs, it is possible that you will not have enough energy for performing your strength training and cardiovascular exercises with 100% effort.

The one thing you can do is practice "Carb Cycling." "Carb Cycling" is simply alternating between low carb days and high carb days.

For example, if you are planning to run 7 miles today, then you would simply eat more carbohydrates today in order to have sufficient energy for your workout.

However, if you were planning to REST tomorrow and not do any exercise, you would then simply keep your carbohydrate intake low in order to prevent storing any excess calories from eating too many carbohydrates.

Keep in mind that both Intermittent Fasting and the Ketogenic Diet are great for controlling your weight and reducing fat loss.

In addition, combining strength training exercises with cardiovascular exercise will help you succeed at developing a body like an ancient Greek warrior.

You have already learned how strength training and cardiovascular exercise will help you to build strength and burn fat.

What I want to talk about now is a unique training method that can be used as a form of cardiovascular exercise.

This unique training method is called **Circuit Training**.

Circuit training is a method of training that requires you to perform one exercise after another with very little to no rest.

For example, look at the following Circuit Training Routine:

<u>**Bodyweight Circuit Routine**</u>
1. Bodyweight squats
2. Pushups
3. Bodyweight lunges
4. Pullups
5. Sit-ups
6. *rest 1 minute and repeat circuit 4 more times*

As you can see from this **Bodyweight Circuit Routine**, you are performing one bodyweight exercise immediately after another.

In addition, circuit training can be performed using machines, medicine balls, dumbbells and barbells.

Here are some other benefits of Circuit Training:
1. Works a lot of different muscles in the body.
2. Burns a lot of calories.
3. Provides a full body workout.
4. Allows you to exercise more in a short amount of time.
5. Develops strength and endurance.
6. Is fun and challenging.

What is great about **Circuit Training** is that you can perform between 4 through 8 **(4-8)** different exercises so that you can work different muscles of the body and get a total body workout.

In addition, you can perform between 6 through 12 **(6-12)** repetitions for each exercise when performing a **Circuit Training** routine.

This number of repetitions will help you to develop strength and improve your stamina as you aim to develop a lean, functional body like the ancient Greeks.

Here are a few more Circuit Training Routines you can use as a guide:

Dumbbell Circuit Routine I
1. Dumbbell deadlifts (6-12 Repetitions)
2. Dumbbell military press (6-12 Repetitions)
3. Dumbbells bent over rows (6-12 Repetitions)
4. Dumbbell squats (6-12 Repetitions)

rest 1 minute and repeat circuit 4 more times

Bodyweight Circuit Routine II
1. Pull-ups (6-12 Repetitions)
2. Jump Rope for 1 minute
3. Parallel Chest Dips (6-12 Repetitions)
4. Jump Rope for 1 minute

rest 1 minute and repeat circuit 4 more times

Bodyweight Circuit Routine III
1. Pull-up burpees (6-12 Repetitions)
2. Use Rowing machine for 1 minute
3. Dumbbell squat to shoulder press (6-12 Repetitions)
4. Use Rowing machine for 1 minute

rest 1 minute and repeat circuit 4 more times
**Alternate running in place or jump roping if there is no available rowing machine.*

It is important to state that starting a cardiovascular exercise routine, whether it is aerobic or anaerobic, is not difficult to do.

All you have to do is simply start off slow.

For example, if you want to start a running routine you can begin doing so by simply running at a slow to medium pace for 10 minutes, 4 days a week.

The following week you would then increase your running routine to 15 minutes, 4 days a week.

You can continue to slowly increase your running mileage until you feel comfortable enough to change up your running routine by doing some sprints.

By first running at a slow to moderate pace, which is consider **aerobic exercise**, you will be developing endurance.

After you have established a good running foundation, you can switch to running sprints, which is considered **anaerobic exercise**.

Remember, **anaerobic exercise** is great for developing strength, speed and power.

By performing both aerobic and anaerobic exercise, you will be developing endurance, strength and speed.

Overall, you will become more athletic and functional as a result of performing both aerobic and anaerobic exercise.

It is important to state that you want to start slow and increase your intensity slowly when beginning the process of doing aerobic and anaerobic exercises.

By starting slow and slowly increasing the intensity of your exercises, you will greatly reduce your chances of getting injured while exercising.

One final point to mention regarding cardiovascular exercise is **CONSISTENCY**.

Consistency is not only important with your cardiovascular exercises but also with your strength training exercises.

Consistency with your workouts is important because you want to continue to burn fat, get lean, improve with your workouts and remain motivated for achieving your health and fitness goals.

Keep this in mind, the minute you begin to skip a workout is the moment you develop the **HABIT** of making it ok to be inconsistent with your workouts.

In addition, being inconsistent with your workouts and simply foolishly skipping workouts can lead to a loss of motivation as well as a loss of strength and endurance which can lead to injury.

It is important to state that if you truly want to develop the physique like an ancient Greek warrior then you have to stay committed to living a health and fitness lifestyle.

Let me tell you, it is rewarding to achieve the body you want especially if you dedicate so much time, effort and discipline with your workouts and eating habits.

Developing a body like the ancient Greeks is something that not many people are willing to do because they are not willing to make a **Commitment** for doing so.

If you think about it, it is actually a lot easier to be **Average** and look like everyone else.

But ask yourself, "Do you want to be average?" "Do you want to look like everyone else?"

Some people may say that striving to develop a physique like the ancient Greeks is all about vanity but it is more, it is a lot more.

Through this process of developing your body, you will also be developing your **MIND**.

In addition, you will learn more about yourself then never before.

You will learn discipline, commitment, focus, sacrifice, determination, resilience, consistency, pain, suffering and achievement.

Now, it may take you 3, 6, 9 months or 1 year to achieve your lean, functional physique but you will achieve it if you are committed to achieving this goal and if you are consistent throughout the process.

In the end, when everything is said and done, you will have the body that you have been longing for.

Chapter 6: Your 8-Week Weight Training Guide

Before we begin, it is important to state that everybody will have a different starting point when it comes to beginning a weight training program.

As a result, it is important to tailor your weight training program according to your fitness levels.

The following weight training guide combines both strength training exercises as well as cardiovascular exercises.

Week one begins with half hour workouts that are meant to progress as weeks go on.

If you feel that starting with shorter workouts is better for your current fitness levels, then go ahead and cut the workouts in half.

The idea for the weight training program is for you to slowly progress and get stronger based on your current fitness levels.

In addition, you want to keep in mind that your weight training goal is to get stronger than you currently are and not to compete with others.

It is important to state that all the exercises that you will be performing for the weight training program will target all the muscle groups in the body.

In addition, be aware of any previous injuries you may have suffered and make sure to modify the weight training program as needed.

Remember you want to always think safety first when it comes to exercise.

As you look over the weight training program you will notice that there are only workouts scheduled for four or five days of the week.

The reason there are only workouts scheduled for four or five days of the week is because **Rest** and **Recovery** are very important in order for the body to repair itself and to avoid injury.

Actually, in the beginning you may even want to go ahead and modify the weight training program by resting more but it is important that you remain consistent with your training.

As stated before, tailor your weight training program according to your fitness levels.

Also, pay attention to how your body feels and if you feel your body needs more rest, then don't hesitate to take an extra day of rest.

Keep in mind that if you do rest more, this does not mean that you should simply sit down all day and do nothing.

Instead, you want to continue to exercise your heart and body by doing some easy exercise like walking.

Keep in mind that all weight training and weight bearing exercises are meant to be done slowly.

When performing an exercise, you want to make sure you take your time performing the exercise, have good form and really put in the necessary work for getting a great workout.

Week One: Determine your Baseline and Warm-up

This first week should be dedicated to finding out what your fitness levels are. You want to simply test your overall strength, agility and flexibility with various exercises.

Let's begin.

Week 1

You want to begin by doing a strength training workout on **day one**.

Then on **day two** you will do a cardiovascular workout.

Then on **day three** you will rest and recover.

So, you will follow this training schedule in the following order:
1. Day One – Strength Training
2. Day Two – Cardiovascular Workout
3. Day Three - Rest and Recover

Repeat this workout schedule routine, day after day, following the exact order throughout the entire 8-week training schedule.

Warm-up

You want to begin every strength training session with a 5-10-minute warm-up.

A warm-up can consist of the following body movements:

<u>**Warm-up Routine**</u>
1. Arm circles

2. Shoulder rotations
3. Neck circles
4. Waist rotations
5. Leg swings
6. 5-10 repetitions of Jumping jacks
7. Jog in place for 10-30 seconds
8. Feet shuffle side to side like a boxer for 10-30 seconds

repeat warm-up routine 2 to 3 times or as needed.

Here is your strength training workout routine for Week 1:

Strength Training Routine

1. Pushups
2. Bodyweight squats
3. Inverted rows or Chin-ups
4. Dumbbell Shoulder press (use light dumbbells)
5. Bodyweight Lunges

Rest for 1 minute and repeat the workout 4 more times
**Perform 6-12 repetitions for all exercises*

Here is your cardio workout for Week 1:
Cardio Routine

1. First, run or jog on a treadmill for 10 minutes
2. Next, ride a stationary bike for 10 minutes
3. Then, use a rowing machine for 10 minutes

Alternate between an elliptical machine or jump roping if an exercise machine is not available.

Here is how your workout schedule will look Monday through Sunday for Week 1:

Monday	Tuesday	Wednes-day	Thursday	Friday	Saturday	Sunday
Strength Training Routine	Cardio Routine	***Rest and Recovery***	Strength Training Routine	Cardio Routine	***Rest and Recovery***	Strength Training Routine

As you can see from this training schedule, you will train two days consecutively which consists of one day of strength training followed by a second day of cardio exercise.

The third day is your rest and recovery day. On your rest day, you can do some "light" exercise like walking.

You will repeat this training cycle for the entire 8-week training program.

It is important to state that overworking your muscles can lead to decreased performance over time, extreme soreness and tiredness and can even lead to injury.

As a result, you can always modify the training schedule but remember to remain consistent with your workouts.

Weeks 2 and 3: Increase Intensity of Week One

Very simply, you will slowly increase the intensity of your workouts from week one by making the exercises more challenging.

In addition, there will be some new strength and cardio exercises included as part of your training for Weeks 2 and 3.

Remember to always warm-up before you begin your strength training routine.

Here is your strength training workout for Weeks 2 and 3:

Strength Training Routine

1. Decline Pushups   (Place both feet on a chair or bench and perform pushups)
2. Goblet squats (Use light weight)
3. Pull-ups   (Alternate between Pull-ups and Chin-ups)
4. Dumbbell shoulder press   (use light to moderate weight)
5. Dumbbell Lunges (use light weight)

Rest for 1 minute and repeat the workout 4 more times
Perform 6-12 repetitions for all exercises

Here is your cardio workout for Weeks 2 and 3:

Cardio Routine

1. First, jump rope for 10-15 minutes
2. Then, use a rowing machine for 10-15 minutes
3. Next, use an elliptical machine for 10-15 minutes

Alternate between a treadmill or stationary bike if an exercise machine is not available.

Here is how your workout schedule will look Monday through Sunday for Weeks 2 and 3:

Monday	Tuesday	Wednes-day	Thursday	Friday	Saturday	Sunday
Strength Training Routine	Cardio Routine	*Rest and Recovery*	Strength Training Routine	Cardio Routine	*Rest and Recovery*	Strength Training Routine

Continue to follow your workout schedule of strength training day one, followed by doing cardio on day two, followed by resting on day three then repeating the cycle all over again on day four.

Continue to follow this workout schedule to make sure you build sustainable strength, stamina and for allowing your body to get enough rest.

Remember to do some "light" exercise on your "rest days" like walking.

Weeks 4 and 5: New Exercises and More Intensity

You will continue to increase the intensity of your workouts from the previous weeks by performing new exercises as well as increasing the intensity of your workouts.

In addition, you will perform "superset" routines for your strength training workouts.

"Supersets" are exercises that work opposing muscle groups. For example, chest and back exercises performed one right after the other are considered a "superset."

In addition, "Supersets" can also be exercises that work the upper and lower body by performing one exercise immediately after the other.

For example, performing a set of pushups for the upper body then immediately performing a set of bodyweight squats for the lower body will be considered a "superset."

Because you will be performing new exercises, you will be using some extra equipment in order to further challenge yourself as you progress with your workouts.

Here is your strength training workout for Weeks 4 and 5:

Strength Training Superset Routine I
1. Weighted Chin-ups   (Use Light Weight)
2. Explosive Jumping squats (Use 100% effort)

Rest for 1 minute and repeat the workout 4 more times
**Perform 6-12 repetitions for all exercises*

Strength Training Superset Routine II
1. Parallel Dips Exercise
2. Reverse Dumbbell Lunges (use light to moderate weight)

Rest for 1 minute and repeat the workout 4 more times
**Perform 6-12 repetitions for all exercises*

Strength Training Superset Routine III
1. Dumbbell Shoulder Push Press   (use light to moderate weight)
2. Mountain Climbers   (use bodyweight)

Rest for 1 minute and repeat the workout 4 more times
**Perform 6-12 repetitions for all exercises*

Here is your cardio workout for Weeks 4 and 5:

Cardio Routine I
1. Perform Stair Running (Run up and down a flight of stairs for 30 seconds)

Rest for 1 minute and repeat the workout 10 more times
* Alternate Running every step, then running every other step.*

Cardio Routine II
    1. First use a rowing machine for 10-15 minutes
    2. Next, use an elliptical machine for 10-15 minutes
Alternate between a treadmill or stationary bike if an exercise machine is not available.

Weeks 6 and 7: Developing Strength, Endurance and Athleticism

By now, you should have developed some strength, speed, balance, agility, coordination, conditioning and flexibility.

Now you will continue to develop your strength, endurance and overall athleticism with more new and intense exercises.

Here is your strength training workout for Weeks 6 and 7:

Strength Training Routine I
    1. Dumbbell Renegade Rows to Mountain Climbers (Use Light Weight)
Rest for 1 minute and repeat the workout 4 more times
**Perform 6-12 repetitions*

Strength Training Routine II
    1. Dumbbell squat to shoulder press (Use Light Weight)
Rest for 1 minute and repeat the workout 4 more times
**Perform 6-12 repetitions*

Strength Training Routine III
    1. Pushups to Pull-ups Burpee
Rest for 1 minute and repeat the workout 4 more times
**Perform 6-12 repetitions*

Here is your cardio workout for Weeks 6 and 7:

Cardio Routine I
1. Perform Stair Running Carrying light dumbbells or weights for 30 seconds

Rest for 1 minute and repeat the workout 10 more times
**Alternate Running every step, then running every other step.*

Cardio Routine II
1. Perform 30 to 60-second Rowing Sprints

Rest for 1 minute and repeat the workout 10 more times
Alternate between a treadmill or stationary bike if an exercise machine is not available.

Cardio Routine III
1. Use an elliptical machine for 10-15 minutes

Alternate between a treadmill or stationary bike if an exercise machine is not available.

Week 8: Test Yourself

You have come so far with your training. Now it is time to TEST your physical abilities.

It is important to state that the following tests only test a few specific exercises.

So, what you can do is test yourself using additional exercises if you like but simply use the following tests as a guide.

Keep in mind that before you test yourself, you want to make sure you properly warm-up.

In addition, you want to give yourself a few minutes to rest in between tests.

Here are the following tests you can use to measure your physical abilities:

Test #1 Pull-ups
You want to test yourself to see how many **pull-ups** you can do without stopping. Make sure to go all out and do your best!

Test #2 Parallel Dips Exercise
You want to test yourself to see how many **parallel dips** you can do without stopping. Make sure to go all out and do your best!

Test #3 Run 3 Miles for Time
You want to test yourself to see how **fast** you can **run 3 miles**. Use a stop watch to time yourself. In addition, make every effort to run as **fast** as possible.

After you complete the three tests determine if you need to improve your fitness levels.

If you realize that you do need to improve your fitness levels than simply retest yourself in 3 or 4 weeks.

One thing to keep in mind is that you always want to be improving with your workouts.

In addition, don't always do the same exercises and workouts months after months.

Instead, always be "evolving" with your workouts by trying new exercises and challenging yourself with new training equipment as well.

One final point I want to mention before we move on to the next chapter is the importance of stretching.

Stretching after you finish exercising whether it is completing a strength training session or a cardio workout is extremely important for the human body.

The kind of stretching you want to do after completing a tough workout is called "static stretching."

"Static stretching" is stretching a part of your body and holding this stretch for 30 seconds or more.

For example, holding onto a pull-up bar and hanging for 30 seconds would be considered "static stretching."

Another example of "static stretching" would be sitting down on the floor and reaching forward to touch your toes and holding this position for 30 seconds or more.

Here are some benefits of static stretching:
1. Improves your flexibility and the body's range of motion.
2. Reduces muscle soreness.
3. Corrects muscle imbalances of the joints.
4. Reduces risk of injury.
5. Improves athletic performance.

As you can see, stretching after completing a workout is very important for the body.

Try to do between 10 and 15 minutes of stretching after working out in order to "cool down" and relax the body and mind.

Chapter 7: Ancient Greek Nutrition

Working out hard is important and easy to do.

But what is very difficult for many people to do is to properly fuel their bodies with the right foods.

In order to perform at your best when working out, you have to eat the right foods in order to properly fuel your body.

In addition, in order to burn fat, get lean and build muscle you have to discipline yourself to follow a healthy eating plan.

Because you want to build a lean functional physique like the ancient Greeks, let's look at nutrition through the eyes of the ancient Greeks themselves.

For example, the ancient Greeks ate bread dipped in wine for breakfast whereas modern day breakfast consists of drinking sugary juice and eating bacon and maybe some eggs or a bagel.

For lunch the ancient Greeks would eat more bread dipped in wine but it also included eating dried fish, olives, figs and cheese.

For the ancient Greeks, dinner was the main meal of the day consisting of fish, vegetables and fruit.

To give their food some flavor, the ancient Greeks would use natural honey as a way to sweeten their food.

The ancient Greeks were known to eat a lot of fish. In addition, fish was the main source of protein for the ancient Greeks.

However, the amount of fish and meat an ancient Greek person would eat would depend on how wealthy they were.

Beef was rarely eaten because it was very expensive and pork was eaten by poor Greeks and slaves.

It is important to state that the ancient Greeks ate very little meat especially when you compare how much meat is consumed every day in developed nations.

The ancient Greeks were considered "frugal" with their food. Only the wealthy would indulge in eating lots of meat and beef.

The ancient Greeks were known for consuming a lot of wine. However, the wine would be "watered down" and was consumed slowly.

Milk was not consumed by the ancient Greeks but instead it was used for producing cheese.

Because the ancient Greeks did not have forks, spoons or knives to use for eating, they would simply eat with their hands.

In addition, the ancient Greeks would use bread to eat their soup by scooping it up using the bread.

It can be said that the ancient Greeks ate a lot of bread and the two main grains they used for making bread were wheat and barley.

For the ancient Greeks, fruits and vegetables were a very important part of their diet.

The ancient Greeks would include a lot of vegetables in their soups. In addition, foods like lentil soup were very popular with the ancient Greeks.

An everyday working Greek man would eat a lot of lentil soup and garlic and a Greek soldier's main source of food consisted of onions and cheese.

Fruits and nuts were eaten as desserts. The most important fruits for the ancient Greeks were pomegranates, raisons and dried figs.

Ancient Greek warriors like the Spartans would mostly eat a "black soup" or "black broth" made up of boiled pork, pig's blood, vinegar and salt.

This "black soup" the Spartans would eat was a staple food for them because they believed it would give them extreme strength and power.

In addition, this "black soup" the Spartans would eat was served with dried figs and cheese and if they were lucky, sometimes they would get to eat some fish or other animal.

Now those Greeks that lived along the coastline would eat a lot of fresh fish and seafood.

In addition, foods like sardines and anchovies were very popular with those Greeks that lived along the coastline.

Another important food the ancient Greeks would eat were eggs.

Greeks ate eggs specifically from hens and quails. In addition, eggs were often eaten as appetizers or dessert.

Another important food that was a staple food for the ancient Greeks was cheese.

Cheese was often eaten with honey and vegetables.

In addition, nuts like walnuts and almonds were very popular with the ancient Greeks.

And when it comes to water, the ancient Greeks would drink a lot of "spring water" which was always preferred over water from wells.

After water, wine was their drink of choice. The ancient Greeks would sometimes sweeten their wine with honey.

There were also religious Greeks that practiced vegetarianism with some Greeks restricting themselves to only eating bread and water.

Ancient Greeks would also use a lot of herbs in their cooking and meals.

The ancient Greeks did not complicate their meals but instead simply ate what was available to them.

Now that you know a little about what the ancient Greek people used to eat, lets focus now on what the ancient Greek Athletes used to eat.

Greek Athletes

Ancient Greek athletes ate simple foods. If they could afford it, they would eat meat but fish was the preferred source of protein for Greek athletes.

In addition, Greek athletes ate a lot of dried fruit. For example, dried figs were a main source of food for the ancient Greek athletes.

Greek athletes would practice the importance of having a healthy diet especially if they were to participate in the Olympic Games.

Usually, an athlete's diet would consist of foods such as fresh cheese, bread and dried figs.

Some athletes were even instructed to eat more meat and follow a "meat diet" which consisted of eating a lot of meat for the purpose of getting stronger.

For example, there was this very famous Olympic champion wrester that was considered to be the greatest wrestler of ancient Greece.

He was known to eat 20 pounds of meat per day! In addition, he would eat several pounds of bread every day as well as drink lots and lots of wine on a daily basis.

Now this ancient Greek wrestler was the exception and not the norm.

But overall, Greek athletes were known for eating a healthy balanced diet and they were very careful about the foods they ate.

Greek athletes also had trainers that would teach them about the importance of having a healthy diet.

For example, athletic trainers would instruct the Greek athletes to stay away from desserts and from drinking wine.

Greek athletes would also eat bread, specifically flatbread which was made of barley or wheat.

Although the amount of wine a Greek athlete would consume during training was reduced or eliminated, they still enjoyed consuming their wine.

In addition, Greek athletes loved olive oil.

It can be said that Greek athletes truly enjoyed consuming olive oil so much that some athletes went as far as bathing themselves in olive oil before a fitness competition.

It is important to mention that just as there are different food diets and food trends today, there were also food trends during ancient Greece times.

For example, if there was a Greek athlete that stated he did not eat bread for whatever reason, then other people would soon follow this "no bread" diet.

Another food trend that was popular with Greek athletes was the "raw honey" diet.

There were some Greek athletes that believed that consuming lots of raw honey would give them lots of energy for making them top performing athletes.

However, after some years, other Greek athletes would practice the "no honey" diet because they believed the sugar in honey would make them slow.

What is interesting about these food trends during ancient Greece was that Greek athletes were not looking for a food trend to follow but instead they were seeking to improve their diets with a sense of "perfection" and "purity."

It can be said that the diet of ancient Greek athletes was simple consisting of fish, bread, olive oil and wine.

However, the Greek athletes placed great importance on eating the best and purest sources of food that would help them to succeed in their sport and in the Olympic Games.

As you can recall from the previous chapters, the ancient Greeks believed a lot in "perfection."

The Greek athletes wanted to eat the perfect foods and have the perfect diet and the Greeks in general believed in having ideal perfect physiques.

Even the Greek statues were created with great perfection by its sculptors.

Even the Greek farmers strived to grow perfect crops for the athletes and for the general Greek population to eat.

The ancient Greeks were definitely perfectionists.

Food and The Olympic Games

Before we continue to learn more about Greek athletes and their eating habits let's look at a brief history regarding the Olympic Games:
1. Ancient Olympia is the birthplace of the Olympic Games.
2. The first Olympic Games were held in 776 B.C.
3. The Olympic Games were meant to honor Zeus, the God of Sky and Thunder and King of the Gods.
4. Only men were allowed to attend and watch the Olympic Games.

It is important to state that Greek athletes that were participating in the Olympic games were required to travel long distances by foot or sea to the small city village of Olympia.

Because the village of Olympia was so small, it did not have enough food to feed all the athletes as well as all the people that would go to watch the Olympic Games.

So, many athletes, with the help of farmers, would package nothing but the best and healthiest foods and carry this food with them to the Olympic Games.

The Greek athletes were also required to bring enough food to last the long journey to the Olympic Games from their hometowns.

The Greek athletes also had to bring enough food to eat during the Olympic Games.

They Greek athletes also had to bring enough food to eat for the giant celebration that followed the conclusion of the Olympic Games.

And the Greek athletes still had to make sure they had enough food for their trip back to their hometowns after the Olympic Games were over.

As you can see, the ancient Greeks were not only athletes but also true warriors.

It can be said that Greek athletes developed a mental toughness mindset of surviving on little food yet competing at the highest levels in sports competition for honor and glory.

Because the Olympic Games and training as an athlete for the Olympic Games were very important, the farmers were always making sure to grow the best foods for the Greek athletes.

In addition, the farmers made every effort to prepare food for the Greek athletes well in advanced for the Olympic Games.

In addition, the farmers were very proud of the foods they grew for the Greek athletes.

The farmers believed that if a Greek athlete was victorious at the Olympic Games it was because they were growing the best foods.

What can be said of ancient Greek athletes is that they spent years perfecting their diets as well as transporting their food from their hometowns to the Olympic Games.

With the help of farmers, Greek athletes made sure to eat nothing but the best foods they could feed their bodies.

And if Greek athletes were to become victorious during the Olympic Games, it was because of the foods they ate.

Now that you know a little about what ancient Greek athletes ate to perform at their highest levels, let's look at how you too can eat like an ancient Greek athlete.

Eating Like the Ancient Greeks

It has been said that if you want to be successful at something, do what successful people do.

So, if you want to develop a lean, functional physique like the ancient Greeks then simply eat and train like the ancient Greeks.

Exercising and training especially in modern times is very easy to do because we have access to all kinds of gyms, fitness equipment, online exercise videos and fitness apps to help us with our workouts.

But the hard part of developing a lean, functional physique is not the exercise part but rather following a healthy diet every day for 3, 6, 9 months or 1 year.

If you can practice eating a healthy diet every day for several months than you will be successful at developing an athletic physique like the ancient Greeks.

What is important to remember is that developing a lean functional physique like the ancient Greeks is all about living a health and fitness lifestyle.

Therefore, you have to make living a health and fitness lifestyle a **priority** in your life if you truly want to develop a lean, functional physique.

You already learned that following a healthy diet for the ancient Greeks was very important.

Therefore, it is going to be just as important for you to also follow a healthy diet especially now more than ever because of the easy access we have to processed and unhealthy foods.

You want to always keep in mind to do as the ancient Greeks did and that is to keep your diet simple and focus on eating natural healthy foods.

Consider the following foods for eating simple, natural, healthy foods:

1. For eating healthy sources of protein, focus on eating fish and chicken.

2. For eating vegetables, consider eating spinach, lettuce and broccoli.

3. For eating healthy carbohydrates, consider eating legumes and sweet potatoes.

4. For eating healthy fats, consider eating avocados and healthy nuts like almonds and walnuts.

5. To add flavor to your food, consider using lemon, spicy hot sauce or some low calorie sweet sauce.

As you can see from this simple but natural food list, eating healthy does not have to be difficult.

You just have to make a commitment to eating healthy followed by creating a plan regarding the types of foods you plan to eat.

Chapter 8: Health Benefits of Eating and Training Like the Ancient Greeks

The goal of eating and training like the ancient Greeks is not just to have a great body, but to live a healthier life.

In addition, by eating natural healthy foods and making exercise part of your daily life, you will be 10 times healthier than the majority of people.

It is important to state that by developing a naturally lean and powerful body like the ancient Greeks, you will develop confidence and discipline within yourself.

In addition, you will come to know what pain and sacrifice are.

You will develop mental toughness and a winning mindset to succeed at achieving your goals.

You will develop tremendous patience and focus especially in a time when everyone wants to lose 10 pounds in 1 day.

Let me tell you this journey of developing a lean, functional physique is not going to be easy nor fast but the process and the end goal are well worth it.

It can be stated that after several months of staying committed to eating healthy and training hard, you will feel victorious just like the ancient

Greek athletes felt victorious when they succeeding at winning at the Olympic Games.

It is important to state that going through the process of developing a lean, functional physique is an excellent goal to achieve but what is more important is what you will become as a result of achieving this goal.

You will become a "role model" to others of how to live, eat and train like a modern-day warrior.

People will look up to you and ask you about how they too can achieve their health and fitness goals.

Remember, you are not seeking to be a bodybuilder but instead you are seeking to develop a lean, functional physique.

It is important to state that many people are looking for "shortcuts" to achieving their health and fitness goals by taking all kinds of supplements, steroids and other stimulants.

However, it is very important that you stay away from all of these supplements and stimulants and remain "natural" because all of those supplements and stimulants will negatively affect your overall health later in life.

Keep in mind that the idea of creating an ideal Greek body is all about achieving good health the natural way.

In order to benefit from eating healthy and training like the ancient Greeks, you must truly embrace this lifestyle

Keep in mind that the ancient Greeks lived in a very different time than we currently live in today.

The ancient Greeks lived in an era before there were so many modern conveniences like easy access to all kinds of foods, supermarkets and fast food restaurants that deliver food in 30-minutes or less.

In addition, the ancient Greeks were a lot busier than people are today.

For example, there was no time for a Greek person to sit around and surf the internet, watch television or play video games because computers and televisions had not yet been invented.

Instead, the ancient Greeks were active in their communities as well as busy working as farmers or they would simply be out enjoying nature.

There were also those ancient Greeks that stayed busy by training religiously to be soldiers, warriors and Olympic athletes.

Should you decide to embrace the ancient Greek lifestyle and live with the purpose of creating a body that is both healthy and functional, your health and overall quality of life will greatly improve.

If you need more reasons to embrace the ancient Greek warrior lifestyle then consider the following 11 benefits of living this amazing lifestyle:

1. Regular exercise and eating healthy both improve your mood and give you tremendous energy.
2. Exercise and eating healthy fight off diseases and illnesses and prevent obesity.
3. Exercise and healthy eating improve your quality of sleep and extend your lifespan.
4. Exercise and healthy eating improve your levels of productivity at work and in your overall life.
5. Exercise and healthy eating help you to look and feel younger.

6. Eating healthy and physical exercise help you to focus better, improve your memory, make you more alert and improve your brain power making you smarter.
7. Eating healthy and doing exercise will strengthen you heart, body and mind.
8. Exercise and eating healthy will reduce stress and help you to relax more.
9. Eating healthy and physical exercise will improve your confidence and help you to be more creative.
10. Exercise and eating healthy can be fun, social and improve your sex life.
11. Physical exercise and eating healthy can help you to develop discipline, commitment, focus, patience and determination.

As you can see, there are so many benefits of why living a healthy and fitness lifestyle like the ancient Greeks is so rewarding.

Sure, it will be difficult at times especially in the beginning and sure, it will take time to burn some fat and get fit but so what.

Simply, EVERYTHING TAKES TIME!

Make a positive step in your life by committing to living a health and fitness lifestyle for the next eight weeks.

After eight weeks, evaluate your results by asking yourself the following questions:

1. "How much fat did I burn?"

2. "How much stronger did I get?"

3. "How do I feel after eight weeks of living a health and fitness lifestyle?"

4. "How has my quality of life improved?"

Even after eight weeks of training and eating healthy, consider making living a health and fitness lifestyle a permanent goal.

Keep in mind that your health and fitness lifestyle does not have to be perfect but you do have to be consistent with your workouts and with maintaining your healthy eating habits.

Remember, you are human so you will make mistakes along your health and fitness journey.

However, never be discouraged and always remember that you are living a positive and rewarding health and fitness lifestyle the ancient Greek way.

Conclusion

Thanks for making it through to the end of *Bodybuilding: How to Build the Body of a Greek God.*

This book has been about more than just creating the body of a Greek God.

This book has taught you about how the ancient Greeks lived, ate and trained on a daily basis.

This book has also taught you how the ancient Greeks saw the human body as a beautiful art form.

Now that you have come to learn the overall lifestyle that ancient Greek warriors lived in order to achieve their ideal physiques, it is now time for you to go out and live that same lifestyle.

Remember, the ancient Greeks were active members of society. They used brute strength and stamina on a daily basis and developed their lean, athletic bodies without even trying.

In addition, the ancient Greeks followed a very healthy but simple diet that consisted of natural foods they grew and raised themselves.

So, if you are looking to develop a body like a Greek God, then you must learn to adjust your lifestyle to one that supports and maintains your physique.

Hopefully, this book was informative and was able to provide you with all of the tools you need to achieve your goal of developing a lean, functional physique.

Remember, developing a lean, functional physique is a process and it will take hard work and commitment.

Therefore, use the information you have learned in this book and make a commitment to transform your body and your life.

Health and Fitness
Chief Aim

*Use the following guide for achieving your health and fitness goals.

Step #1

Write down your health and fitness goal(s) and be specific. For example, if you want to lose 10 pounds then write down, "I want to lose 10 pounds."

At the same time, if you want to build muscle, be specific and write down the amount of muscle you want to have. For example, if you want to have 10 pounds of muscle then write down, "I want to have 10 pounds of muscle."

Step #2

Write down the date by which you want to achieve your health and fitness goal(s).

For example, "I will lose 10 pounds by February 2019."

Example two, "I will be able to run 15 miles nonstop by May 2019."

Step 3

Write down what you are willing to sacrifice in order to achieve your health and fitness goals. In addition, write down what are you willing to give back (to the world) in return for achieving your health and fitness goal(s).

For example, "I am willing to give up drinking alcohol, specifically beer for the next 3 months in order to lose 20 pounds of fat. In addition, I am going to stop watching television after 10:00 PM and I will instead go to sleep early so that I can wake up early and exercise."

"In return for achieving my health and fitness goals, I will serve as a role model inspiring and helping others to also achieve their health and fitness goals by sharing my knowledge, experience and wisdom."

Step 4

Repeat looking and reading over your Health and Fitness Chief Aim every day until you achieve your health and fitness goals. In addition, look and read over your Health and Fitness Chief Aim multiple times a day. Daily repetition is important for achieving any goal.

STRENGTH TRAINING (SECRETS)

The Best Tips and
Strategies to Getting Stronger

By Epic Rios

"Pour your whole soul into exercises you love to do, disregard those exercises you don't like and you will forever be motivated to achieving your fitness pursuits."

– Epic Rios

Table of Contents

Introduction

Congratulations on purchasing *Strength Training Secrets: The Best Tips and Strategies to Getting Stronger.*

The following chapters will discuss how eating healthy and ensuring you receive plenty of rest is not only beneficial to your body, but also how it affects your strength training regimen.

We will go over the basics of strength training and how to get started if you have never done anything like it before.

This will then lead us into the 5x5 workout and some of the best workouts for your legs, chest, and back.

We will also discuss the king of strength training exercises: The Squats.

After that you will learn about some healthy recipes that are ideal for all your nutritional needs so that you can come up with some meal plans for your exercise program.

There will also be a glossary for some of the terms you may not know so that you are able to easily refer to those words as you work your way through this book.

This book will provide you with detailed instructions for how to do a certain exercise.

You will also be provided with pictures of exercises for each workout so that you are able to visually see how each workout should be properly done.

Thanks again for choosing *Strength Training Secrets: The Best Tips and Strategies to Getting Stronger*!

Every effort was made to ensure it is full of as much useful information as possible. Please enjoy!

Chapter 1: Healthy Eating & Rest

Healthy Eating

10 Foods for Building Muscle Mass

1. Healthy Fats
2. Fruits & Vegetables
3. Whole Grains
4. Oatmeal
5. Tuna & Other Fish
6. Cottage Cheese
7. Eggs
8. Skinless Chicken
9. Whey Protein
10. Lean Beef

When it comes to getting lean and strong, diet is very important. Actually, losing weight is all about having a good strict diet.

As you can see diet is very important whether you want to get strong or lose weight or both.

There is a very simple rule that you can follow when it comes to your diet and it is the **80/20 Rule.**

Simply, **80% of the time** eat healthy and **20% of the time** eat unhealthily.

But if you are talking about sport, athleticism or simply getting lean and strong than diet is very important and the **80/20 Rule** could be changed to the **90/10 Rule** where 90% of the time you eat healthy and 10% of the time you eat unhealthily.

As you go through your strength training journey you have to always make every effort to eat as healthy as possible.

Eating healthy is not only good for our health but eating healthy will provide the body with the proper nutrients it needs for it to get strong.

Eating good quality healthy food affects your daily life.

Eating good quality food provides you with a better quality of life as well as more energy for your workouts.

In addition, eating good quality food provides the body with healthy skin as well as with a properly working digestive system.

It is recommended to eat every 3 hours to keep your metabolism up and to also ensure you are having an adequate intake of calories.

However, new research has shown that intermittent fasting and the ketogenic diet can help you better organize your eating schedule while you still achieve your strength training goals.

When it comes to strength training, the goal is to gain muscle, burn fat and get lean.

As you progress with your strength training workouts, you will get stronger and develop more muscle that will replace unwanted fat.

In addition, if you practice a combination of intermittent fasting and the ketogenic diet, you will also feel less hungry throughout the day as you will have a set eating schedule that will be suitable to your strength training schedule.

By combining both intermittent fasting and the ketogenic diet with strength training, you will replace smaller meals with larger meals which will eventually shrink your stomach and get you lean.

If you combine both intermittent fasting and the ketogenic diet with strength training, you will also have fewer cravings because your body will become conditioned to a set eating schedule which will prevent you from snacking throughout the day.

In addition, your body will become conditioned to only eating certain foods as a result of following the ketogenic diet's model of eliminating certain foods.

So, say you generally wake up at 7:00 AM. You would simply skip breakfast and have an eating window from say, 11:00 AM to 7:00 PM.

You would be able to eat an early lunch, then maybe have a snack around 3:00 PM and then have dinner at 6:30 PM.

You can also skip the snack and do a good strength training workout around 3:00 PM.

The choice is really up to you to decide what eating schedule is good for you and what time you want to do your strength training workout.

For many years, people have thought that eating a nice healthy breakfast early in the morning was very important for optimal performance.

However, research continues to show that eating breakfast is not important.

In addition, research has also shown that if you do exercise early in the morning while you are fasting, you will burn more calories than if you would of ate breakfast and then gone to the gym to exercise.

It is important to state that you do have to experiment with working out while fasting but if you do feel you need some energy before your workout, you can always workout after your first meal.

When it comes to building lean muscle, it is important to eat protein rich foods like chicken, beef, eggs and fish.

But you also want to make sure to eat some complex carbohydrates so that you can have energy for your workouts.

Some good sources of complex carbohydrates are steel cut oats, sweet potatoes and quinoa or brown rice.

One example of a good morning or afternoon meal is to have an omelet.

The omelet can be packed with not only protein from the eggs, but you can add lean beef in it as well for a boost in protein.

You can also add veggies to your omelet which will make your meal have an added nutrition boost.

You can also include a small bowl of steel cut oats with some berries.

This meal will definitely give you all the energy you need for an afternoon workout.

In order to get stronger, you have to make sure you get the proper nutrients your body needs.

In addition, you have to make sure you are eating protein with every meal because your muscles require protein in order for them to grow.

Something that a lot of people don't know is that protein helps with losing fat because it has a high thermic effect on the body.

Now you are probably wondering how much protein intake you should have a day.

Depending on how much of an active lifestyle you have, the rule of thumb is that you should consume 1 gram of protein for every pound that you weigh.

For example, if you have 4 strength training sessions per week and you weigh 180 pounds, you should consume 180 grams of protein.

Some people tend to consume more protein than is required. However, research show that if you consume too much protein, it may be stored as fat.

A lot of people that are into strength training tend to drink a lot of protein shakes in order to feed their muscles the required protein their bodies need.

However, it is far healthier to eat whole natural foods that contain good amounts of protein like beef, chicken and fish.

When you eat whole natural protein rich foods your body will feel full as a result of having to breakdown the foods in order for them to be digested.

However, if you drink a protein shake, you will not feel full. Instead, you will feel hungry and you will still need to eat whole natural foods in order to stay full.

The next thing you want to make sure of is that you are eating fruits and vegetables with every meal you eat.

Actually, you want to eat more vegetables than fruits but you do want to include some good nutritious fruits with your meals.

It is important to state that most fruits and vegetables are low in calories and you can eat them until you have a full stomach.

However, fruits tend to have sugar in them and some of them have more sugar then others.

Therefore, you want to eat fruits that have very little sugar like avocado's, blueberries, blackberries, raspberries.

It is important to state that fruits and vegetables are jam packed with things that are good for you such as antioxidants, vitamins and minerals, and even fiber which aids your body in digestion.

It is also important to state that without consuming the proper amount of digestive enzymes, your body will actually break down tissues.

This includes muscle tissue which you do NOT want to do.

As a result, it is crucial for bodybuilders and anyone else who is looking to gain muscle mass to include plenty of foods in their diet that contain digestive enzymes.

This means staying away from processed foods as they do not have any nutritional value.

In addition, processed foods do not have digestive enzymes as a result of the manner in which they are prepared.

That is why it is better to eat whole natural foods so that you can get the proper enzymes and nutrients your body needs.

If people who are trying to gain muscle pay enough attention to their intake of these digestive enzymes and nutrients, they will see far better results than someone who does not.

Another thing to keep in mind is to make sure you eat carbs after your workout.

It is true that many people eat more carbs than they should which is why it is recommended to only eat them after working out.

However, feel free to eat carbs but practice portion control when it comes eating carbs.

If you are skinny and you wish to gain weight, then feel free to eat more carbs than are required but make sure they are healthy carbs like fruits and vegetables.

When it comes to eating carbs, you want to stay away from white carbs and instead eat whole grain foods.

As stated before, some good complex carbohydrates are steel cut oats, sweet potatoes and brown rice or quinoa.

For example, avocados are a fruit but they have healthy fats that are full of fiber and other nutrients and that keep you feeling full longer.

Salmon is also considered a good source of healthy fat.

Nuts, like walnuts, almonds and cashews are also good sources of healthy fats.

The yoke in an egg is also considered a healthy fat.

And instead of using regular cook oil for cooking you can instead use olive oil. Olive oil is a good source of fat and is very popular with the Mediterranean diet.

Now, healthy fats are foods that many people don't know about.

Many people know that there are unhealthy foods that will make you fat but many people are not aware of healthy fatty foods and their benefits.

Healthy fats have so many benefits. They increase fat loss and improve overall health. They also satisfy hunger and they digest slowly, meaning you will stay full longer.

You want to make sure to avoid trans fats like margarine because they will increase your cholesterol levels and are a major cause of heart disease.

In addition, you will want to make sure your healthy fat intake is well balanced with fruits, vegetables, complex carbohydrates and lean protein.

When it comes to getting stronger and building lean muscle mass it is important to eat saturated fats like red meat because saturated fats increase testosterone levels.

In addition, monounsaturated fats such as mixed nuts protect against cancers and fight off heart disease.

Polyunsaturated fats such as those found in fish oil not only increase testosterone but they also decrease inflammation and promote fat loss.

Let's not forget that as you strength train and eat properly making sure to get all the nutrients your body needs, you must remember to drink plenty of water.

The rule of thumb is to consume 1 gallon of water per day or more.

Drinking water not only prevents dehydration but it also keeps you feeling full preventing you from getting hungry so often.

In addition, it is important to replenish any loss of water from sweating during your intense workouts.

One thing to keep in mind is that if you don't drink enough water, you will feel hungry especially if you don't eat.

A good habit to develop is to start the morning or your day by drinking 1 glass of water as soon as you wake up.

By drinking 1 cup of water as soon as you wake up, you can increase your metabolism, you will flush out any toxins from your body and you won't feel hungry in the morning.

In addition, you want to be well hydrated before you exercise because research has shown that many people are always tired as result of not drinking enough water or simply being dehydrated.

Water is the lifeblood of the body so you want to make sure that you don't start getting fatigue during your workouts as a result of dehydration.

You will also want to make sure that you are drinking at least 2 cups of water with every meal.

So, disregard drinking juice or soda with your meals and instead get into the habit of drinking water with all of your meals.

Now that you know a little about what you should be eating here are some sample eating schedules that you can modify according to your strength training workouts and lifestyle:

Schedule 1
Breakfast - egg omelet with veggies, a bowl of steel cut oats and some green tea
Lunch - romaine lettuce salad, 1 or 2 cans of tuna, olives, and olive oil
Dinner - chicken tenders (no skin), spinach and a big sweet potato

Schedule 2 (Intermittent Fasting) (11:00 PM – 7:00 PM)
Early Lunch - chicken breasts with broccoli and mixed veggies, sweet potatoes, 1 whole avocado
3:30 snack - handful of blueberries and handful of walnuts
Dinner - salmon, spinach and a big sweet potato

Schedule 3 (Ketogenic Diet and Intermittent Fasting) (12:00 PM – 8:00 PM)
Lunch - avocado egg omelet and vegetables
3:30 snack - handful of almonds
Dinner - grass fed beef served with avocados and spinach and broccoli veggies

It is important to state that many people nowadays are vegetarian. So, you may be wondering how a vegetarian can possibly get enough protein and hold onto their strength gains.

Chicken, beef and fish are good sources of protein. However, protein can also be found in foods like beans, nuts, legumes, seeds, milk (soy, almond, etc.), veggies and whole grains.

Here is an example of what a vegetarian diet would consist of:
- **Breakfast**- an orange, whole eggs and spinach
- Maybe a Snack- an apple and some mixed nuts/ seeds
- **Lunch-** legumes and a soy burger
- Maybe a Snack- a smoothie that has fruit and veggies with some milk and maybe some whey protein powder
- **Post workout Dinner-** 1 liter of soy or almond milk with a banana or strawberries, tofu and some mixed beans
- Maybe before going to bed – some ground flax seeds, some berries and a serving of cottage cheese

As you can see there is protein in many kinds of foods. So, whether you are a vegetarian or not you have a variety of protein rich foods that you can consume on a daily basis.

Rest

Rest is something many people don't consider when they are thinking about their strength training goals.

For example, many people believe they have to workout quite often, sometimes 5 or 6 times a week, in order to get strong and gain muscle. However, that is not true.

Research shows that the body needs time to recover from a strenuous workout and that resting for a day or two is needed in order for the body to fully recover.

So, in order to be at peak performance when it comes to strength training, you have to be well rested and let your body rest.

Now if you do decide to exercise quite often then your workouts will suffer because you will be forcing your body and muscles to work when they are tired.

In addition, if you do decide to exercise quite often then you may injure yourself as a result of not giving your body the necessary time it needs to recover.

Something that you want to keep in mind is that whenever you do tough strength training exercises, you cause small tears in your muscles.

These tears in the muscles need time to repair and recuperate in order for them to get stronger and grow.

Some people may ask, "What if I exercise different parts of my body each day?"

For example, "What if I exercise my legs on Monday, my chest on Tuesday and my back on Wednesday. Can I do this?"

Well the answer is yes you can exercise different parts of the body day after day.

However, your body will not be functioning at its peak because your entire body will still be recovering from your previous workout.

In addition, your body as a whole still needs to rest in between strength training days because your body's central nervous system is affected whenever you complete a strenuous workout.

Research show that the body's central nervous system is affected after a strenuous strength training workout regardless if only one body part is trained.

In addition, once the body's central nervous system is exhausted from a tough workout, it needs a day or two to recover in order for it to be at its best for the next workout.

So, what this means is that if today you exercised only your legs, your body's central nervous system would be tired and would need time to recover.

Now if tomorrow you went to the gym and tried to train your chest, you may be able to do so.

However, you will not feel as strong because your body's central nervous system will still be tired and recovering from the previous leg workout.

In addition, your body will be sending you messages telling you that it needs more time to rest but you will be forcing your body to exercise because in your mind, you only trained your legs yesterday and so you should be able to exercise a different body part today.

Keep this in mind, when you work out, you are putting stress on your body.

That stress that your body is feeling takes more than 24 hours to recuperate.

Also keep in mind that it is recommended that you give your muscles 48 hours to rest.

This means that you pick a day you want to work out and then you simply go and complete your strength training workout.

Then the following day, you refrain from going to the gym.

Now on the days that you don't go to the gym and that you are resting you can do what's called "active rest."

"Active rest" is exercise that is very low impact as well as light. For example, walking would be considered "active rest" exercise.

So, after a day of completing a tough strength training workout, the following day you can refrain from exercising at the gym and instead do some light walking.

The light walking will be good for your body because you will still be doing some exercise even though it is not strenuous exercise like strength training which causes small tears to your muscles.

Below are some strength training schedules that you can use and modify to fit your training needs:

Sample strength training schedule I
Every other day strength train. In addition, every other day rest.

For example, Sundays, Tuesdays, Thursdays and Saturdays you will strength train.

Then Monday, Wednesday and Friday are your rest days. On your rest days you can do some "light" easy exercise like walking.

Sample strength training schedule II
Every other day do a total body strength training workout.

For example, on Sundays, Tuesdays, Thursdays and Saturdays you will do barbell squats, dumbbell shoulder presses and weighted chin-ups.

Then on Monday, Wednesday and Friday are your rest days. On your rest days you can do some "light" easy exercise like walking.

Sample strength training schedule III
Every other day do a "hybrid" workout.

A "hybrid" workout combines 2 or more exercises for example:
1. barbell squats to shoulder presses
2. pushups to pull-ups
3. pushups to mountain climbers

So, on Sundays, Tuesdays, Thursdays and Saturdays you will do a "hybrid" workout.

Then on Mondays, Wednesdays and Fridays are your rest days. On your rest days you can do some "light" easy exercise like walking.

It is important to state that eating healthy also affects your recovery time, which is something that not many people are familiar with.

Simply you want to give your body the proper nutrients that it needs.

If your body has the proper vitamins and other nutrients it needs, it will have the fuel it needs to recover quickly.

One way to help your body quickly recover from a tough workout is by drinking some chocolate milk immediately after completing a workout.

Chocolate milk has protein and carbs that your body needs in order to rebuild muscle tissue lost during a workout.

If you don't like chocolate milk, you can instead make a chocolate smoothie or simply a banana smoothie with some spinach.

Because the banana smoothie is in liquid form, it will be easier and faster for your body to digest and absorb the nutrients which leads to a faster recovery.

It is important to state that rest isn't all about the rest periods between sets or workouts or even rest days.

Rest is also about the amount of sleep you get every night.

The longer you sleep and the better quality of sleep you have each night the better your recovery will be from strenuous workouts.

Research shows that people who exercise regularly sleep longer and get a better quality of deep sleep.

So, someone who is physically active requires more sleep than a person that does not exercise.

In addition, the more physically active you are, the more sleep you need.

This is because there is more stress on the muscles, the body and the nervous system which means your body needs more time to rest and to rebuild itself.

Many people think that they are getting bigger and stronger when they are strength training.

Instead, what they are doing is actually causing small tears in their muscles.

Now the true growth and muscle building of your muscles takes place while you are sleeping and getting enough rest.

So, the more you exercise, the more rest you will need.

If you do not get an adequate amount of sleep and rest, you may be susceptible to the following:
- Getting sick very easily
- Feeling tired and weak
- Lack of concentration/focus
- Weight gain
- Heart disease, heart attack, and other heart issues.
- Etc.,

As you can see, not getting enough rest and sleep can in turn compromise your health and training.

Another thing to consider when you are training and making sure you are getting enough rest is overtraining.

Overtraining is simply when you exercise too much, too hard and too often without giving your body the necessary rest that it needs.

Overtraining does not occur immediately.

However, as you continue to push through tough workouts day after day, you will begin to feel the effects of overtraining.

Here are some signs of overtraining:
- Extreme soreness
- Loss of appetite
- Tiredness
- Weak immune system

- Etc.,

One side effect of overtraining is the inability to sleep or remain asleep or to simply suffer from insomnia.

If you feel that your sleep is being affected as a result of overtraining, simply tone down your workouts.

Try to exercise every other day with a day of rest in between your workout days.

If you are serious about getting stronger and building more muscle than you will have to develop a schedule and a lifestyle around your training.

So, let's say you want to exercise early in the morning.

That's great! But don't immediately go to the gym and exercise upon waking up because you will still be feeling groggy throughout your workout.

Instead, you want to go to sleep early so that you can wake up early and exercise.

In addition, you want to begin to drink water immediately upon waking up so that you can rehydrate yourself before you go and train.

Trust me when I say this, you will perform better at the gym when you are well hydrated.

One strategy that you can use is too simply wake up 1 hour before going to the gym.

So, if you plan to exercise at 7:00 AM simply wake up at 6:00 AM and begin the process of rehydrating yourself.

Now if you plan to train in the evening, try to do so immediately after work around 5:30 PM.

Research shows that the later you exercise in the evening the harder it will be to go to sleep because your heart rate will be elevated, your body temperature will increase and you will have endorphins giving you energy after your workout making it hard for you to sleep.

In addition, you may be too tired to workout in the evening after a long day of work.

You can always schedule a workout during your lunch break but you have to make sure you plan accordingly.

Keep this in mind, in order to get proper sleep, your body will need to already be somewhat relaxed when you go to bed.

If you are tired or stressed from a good, hard workout, your sleep will suffer.

In addition, you develop a great sense of adrenaline rush with heavy strength training workouts so this is another reason to maybe avoid working out a few hours before you go to sleep.

The bottom line is that your workouts need your full commitment.

So, work on creating a training schedule that is convenient for you and stick to it.

In addition, keep your diet in check.

Above all, make rest and recovery your top priority if you want to get stronger and build lean muscle mass.

Keep this in mind, if for any reason you are unable to get the proper amount of sleep at night, do not hesitate to take a nap during the day.

Research has shown that taking a nap during the day can give you energy, make you feel better as well as increase your overall well-being.

During REM sleep, human growth hormone (HGH) is released.

Human growth hormone is important because it helps maintain healthy body tissue and a healthy metabolism.

In addition, human growth hormone enhances your physical performance and can make you live longer.

So human growth hormone helps the body to repair old and/or malfunctioning cells and basically gives you new life.

Human growth hormone has become very popular in the past few years because of all the benefits it provides.

Human growth hormone can be considered by many to be the "Fountain of Youth" and so many people take human growth hormone supplements or injections in order to look and feel younger.

It is important to state that you can naturally develop human growth hormone by simply doing strength training workouts as well as by getting good quality sleep.

In addition, you can also develop human growth hormone by fasting.

That is why it is important to develop a workout schedule as well as a meal eating schedule so that you can develop a lifestyle around your health and fitness lifestyle.

As you can see, this is why sleep is so important because it will truly help you to live an optimal performing lifestyle.

Now in order to get the best quality of sleep you will need to limit how intense your evening workouts are.

In addition, it would be a good idea to develop an evening ritual for going to sleep.

It is ideal that two hours before bed, you cease any activities that may cause you stress.

Calming ritual behaviors such as brushing your teeth, taking a shower and/or reading a book are ideal for getting good quality sleep.

Another way to make sure that you get in the habit of getting good quality sleep is to create a perfect sleeping environment.

To create a perfect sleeping environment, you can buy curtains that completely block out sunlight.

In addition, you can make sure to close all the windows to make sure that there is no noise coming in from the outside.

You can also regulate the temperature of your bedroom by adjusting the thermostat or simply turning on a fan or heater.

Research show that sleeping in a nice cool bedroom environment will help relax you and help you to fall sleep faster than sleeping in a warm bedroom environment.

You also want to avoid drinking any caffeinated drinks in the evening such as soda and coffee because these beverages will prevent you from going to sleep.

Chapter 2: Training – A Beginner's Guide

Different Types of Strength Training

Bodyweight Exercise: Bodyweight exercises are great because there is little to no equipment needed.

With bodyweight exercises you can exercise anywhere that provides enough room to move around.

Some beginner bodyweight exercises are:
1. Pushups
2. Squats
3. Lunges
4. Sit-ups

Some advance bodyweight exercises are:
1. Pullups or weighted pullups
2. Dips or weighted dips
3. One legged squats also known as Pistols
4. Muscle-ups
5. One hand pushups

There are also exercise bands that you can use to help you with advance exercises like pull-ups, dips and muscle-ups.

It is important to state that many people underestimate just how challenging bodyweight exercises can be.

If you do make bodyweight exercises part of your training it is important to continuously modify your bodyweight exercises to make sure that you are constantly challenging yourself.

In addition, you want to slowly make your bodyweight exercises difficult by using various progressions.

Dumbbells: Dumbbells are great for strength training because there are so many exercises that you can do with them.

For example, you can do:
1. Dumbbell bench press
2. Dumbbell squats
3. Dumbbell rows
4. Dumbbell shoulder presses
5. Dumbbell lunges

First if you train at a gym most gyms have dumbbells so you can easily train with them.

Now if you train at home, there are adjustable dumbbells that you can use that require very little room.

In addition, adjustable dumbbells are a great training tool because the weight can be changed very easily.

Dumbbells are also great because they can be less overwhelming than barbell training and they can help to correct any muscle imbalances that you may have as a result of barbell training.

In addition, dumbbells help to provide more range of motion than barbells.

Barbells: Barbells are perfect for people who want to do traditional barbell exercises like the barbell squat, deadlift and barbell bench press.

Some people believe that only real strength can be developed with barbell exercises.

However, dumbbell exercises are great for developing superior strength and advanced bodyweight exercises like gymnastic exercises develop unbelievable strength with only the use of the human body.

The good thing about barbell training is that barbells are more stable than dumbbells because you must use two hands two lift the weight.

In addition, it is easier to lift heavier weight using a barbell, particularly for lower body exercises like squats or deadlifts.

For example, barbell squats are easy to perform because the barbell is simply placed on the upper part of the back.

In addition, the barbell deadlift is easy to execute because the barbell is simply raised from the ground.

The disadvantage of barbell training is that you need a bench, squat rack, barbell, and enough weights in your garage or house in order to perform exercises like the squat and deadlift.

However, if you have a gym membership, then you will be in luck because most gyms have the required equipment for barbell training.

Which type of training is right for me?

In order to find out which type of strength training is good for you, all you have to do is to simply experiment.

So, if you are someone that likes to train with barbells, simply consider including dumbbells into your training program.

In addition, if you have been into bodyweight exercises for a long time, consider changing up your training by including some barbell and dumbbell exercises into your training.

The truth of the matter is that there is no one best type of training that supersedes the other training methods.

Simply you can get extremely strong with bodyweight, dumbbell or barbell exercises.

It would be smart to use a combination of bodyweight, dumbbell and barbell exercises in order to develop all-around strength as well as to remain motivated with your training program.

Deciding how you want to combine bodyweight, dumbbell and barbell exercises is really up to you.

What is important is that you experiment with your workouts and that you create a training schedule that you can follow.

You can always modify your training schedule but writing down your workouts and organizing them according to your fitness goals is what is extremely important.

Below is a sample workout schedule combing all three types of training:

**Be aware the days that are not listed are rest days

Monday
*Barbell squats
*Barbell bench press
*Wide grip pullups

Wednesday
*Dumbbell shoulder press
*Weighted Chin-ups
*Barbell Deadlift

Friday
*Barbell lunges
*Dumbbell bent over rows
*Bodyweight Dips

Sunday
*Dumbbell squats
*Barbell bent over rows
**Dumbbell bench press

Once you have your training schedule all planned out, it is now time to follow it.

So, for example, if you plan to train early in the morning then you will need to set your alarm clock so that you wake up early.

In addition, you must discipline yourself to sleep early and make the conscious choice that no matter how you are feeling in the morning, you will get up and you will exercise.

After a while, you will not have to even think about going to sleep early and waking up early because you will become accustomed to doing so.

Keep in mind that if you must travel and there are no gyms around, you can always substitute your barbell and dumbbell workouts with bodyweight exercises.

In addition, remember that no matter which type of training you choose a well-balanced, functional body is made by blending all three types of training.

It is important to state that you can also use machines to exercise and get stronger. Other fun ways to do strength training is by rock climbing or doing parkour.

If you are a beginner to strength training you want to look into developing a program that is good for you.

In addition, as a beginner you want to make sure that you slowly increase the intensity and difficultness of your training overtime.

You want to make sure that you try to do better than your previous workouts by doing more repetitions, more workout sets and by slightly adding more weight to your exercises.

This will ensure that you are continually getting stronger as you slowly progress through your workouts.

Keep in mind that at the beginning of every workout you want to always warmup your entire body.

Many people have suffered many injuries as a result of not properly warming up before they exercise.

By warming up the body before you exercise, you will be protecting yourself from injury.

To properly warmup the body you can do what is called "dynamic stretching."

Research shows that "dynamic stretching" is an excellent method for warming up the body before any type of exercise is performed.

Some dynamic stretches that you can do are arm circles, hip rotations and knee raises.

In addition to "dynamic stretching" you can do some light walking or running to warmup the body.

You can also use very light weights to warmup before you exercise and you can even do some very easy bodyweight exercises in order to properly warmup the body.

As your train and continue to excel with your workouts you want to make sure that you keep track of your training schedule and your progress with your workouts.

You want to write down what specific exercises you are going to do and you will include the number of sets and repetitions you will perform as well.

You can also include writing down the amount of weight you will be lifting.

So, you want to develop a plan before you go to the gym and workout and you want to make sure you follow it.

I've heard of overtraining. What is it and how can I avoid it?

Overtraining is when a person does too much exercise which causes a lot of stress on the body and negatively affects training and health.

Sometimes a person overtrains because they are not happy with their fitness results so they tend to do more and more exercise which negatively affects their training and health.

4 Factors That Affect People That Overtrain

The first factor that affects people that overtrain is:

1. **Under-recovering:** Under-recovering is a result of not eating sufficient healthy food as well as not getting enough sleep.

   If you overtrain as well as under-recover you may develop the following symptoms:
   - Anxiety/stress
   - slowed metabolism
   - decrease in your mood
   - suppressed appetite
   - hormonal imbalances
   - missed menstrual cycle
   - sleep disturbances
   - fatigue

   You can prevent overtraining and under-recovery by:
   - sleeping 7-9 hours per night
   - eating plenty of nutritious foods
   - staying away from caffeine and sugar

> ➤ eating slowly so that food can digest properly
> ➤ drink plenty of water
> ➤ varying the intensity of your workouts
> ➤ stretch and work on mobility and other recovery hacks
> ➤ get a massage and seek chiropractic therapy (if needed)
> ➤ take ice baths

2. The second factor that affects people that overtrain is **Work Capacity**.

Work capacity is when you want to do too much too soon and as a result you get injured or are susceptible to injury or overtraining.

For example, sometimes people go to the gym and they lift more weight than they are used to.

In addition, these same people instead of progressing slowly with their training they continue to add too much volume and weight too soon and as a result they end up injuring themselves or they end up overtraining.

When it comes to work capacity, you want to slowly increase your work capacity every week.

In addition, you want to monitor how your body feels after a workout in order to make sure you are not overdoing it with your training.

3. The third factor that affects people that overtrain is **Mindset**. Simply you need to develop the positive mindset to succeed in the gym.

When it comes to strength training many people think they need to exercise more often as well as exercise for 2 or 3 hours in order to get strong and lean. This is simply false.

First you need to educate yourself about how strength training affects the body. In addition, you need to educate yourself about rest and recovery.

You then have to develop discipline to follow through with your training program and develop patience with your training because it will take time for you to see results from all of your hard work.

After you do all this, you will mentally be ready to succeed in the gym and you will most likely avoid overtraining.

But it is important to have the right mindset to succeed in the gym and not let your ego get in the way when it comes to your training.

Simply develop your body by developing your mind. Seek the necessary knowledge that you need to succeed in the gym and with your training and you will definitely avoid overtraining.

4. The fourth factor that affects people that overtrain is **underlying imbalances**.

    Sometimes when a person severely overtrains their entire body is affected.

    For example, some people may suffer from increase weight gain as a result of overtraining.

Some people suffer from fatigue and lack of energy as a result of overtraining.

Some people suffer from anxiety as a result of overtraining.

It is important to state that your current state of health plays a crucial role in your ability to slowly correct any imbalances the body may have.

Rep Ranges and Sample Workouts

People are always wondering what are the best rep ranges or how many repetitions they need to do for getting bigger and stronger.

Below is a brief explanation of the various rep ranges you can use for your training:
  Strength Training Rep Ranges
  ➢ 1-5 reps builds strength and very little size
  ➢ 6-12 reps builds size and some strength
  ➢ 12 reps or more builds muscular endurance and some size

Beginner Bodyweight Workout
  1. 5-10 minute Warm Up (Use Dynamic Stretches)
  2. 10 Bodyweight Squats
  3. 10 Push Ups (If you are unable to do the normal ones, try doing a modified version such as Wall Pushups until you can increase your upper body strength.)
  4. 10 Walking Lunges
  5. 5 jumping pull-ups or Hindu Pushups or suspension rows
  6. Do a 15 second Plank
  7. 30 Jumping Jacks

Repeat Workout 4 times

Here is a popular leg workout consisting solely of squats:

Routine (6-8 Sets)
1. 5-10 minute Warm Up
2. **10 barbell Squats**
3. Rest for 2-3 minutes
4. *Repeat **(6-8 Sets)**

Chapter 3 (5 x 5 Workout)

The 5 X 5 Workout has been popularized by Bill Starr in his book, written in 1976, called "The Strongest Shall Survive: Strength Training for Football."

The 5 x 5 Workout is so effective at building strength that it has been used by top bodybuilders such as Arnold Schwarzenegger.

The 5 X 5 Workout was designed and intended to have the trainee work out hard for 3 days out of the week.

The 5 X 5 workout would then recommend for the trainee to rest the body and muscles the other days of the week in order to ensure proper recovery.

The 5 X 5 Workout's main goal is for a person to develop strength by lifting heavy weight for 5 repetitions 3 times a week and then stimulate muscle growth by allowing the body to rest 4 days a week.

By practicing the 5 X 5 Workout, you will see an increase in muscle mass as long as you eat an adequate amount of calories.

In addition, the low reps, heavy lifting and intensity of the 5 X 5 Workout are very challenging compared to other strength training programs.

So, if you are not used to lifting heavy weights, you will have a hard time recovering from the lifting heavy loads for low repetitions.

However, in the beginning you will go through the process of slowly increasing the weight so that your body can get conditioned to lifting heavy weights for low reps.

The 5 X 5 Workout is a 7-9 weeklong training program.

There are between 4-6 weeks of preparation work followed by 3 weeks of pure, raw, strength training followed by a 1-week deloading phase.

The first part of the 5 X 5 Workout is the preparation phase.

This phase consists of choosing a weight that you can successfully lift for 5 repetitions and for 5 sets.

The weight that you choose to lift for your 5 sets of 5 repetitions should not be easy but instead challenging.

However, you have to make sure that you practice safety first and choose a weight that is challenging for you.

It is important to keep in mind that for the beginning phase of the 5 X 5 Workout, you don't want to feel like the weight that you are lifting is too light.

But at the same time, you don't want the weight to be so heavy that you will not be able to complete your workout.

So, you will have to experiment a little in the beginning to make sure you choose a weight that is challenging for you.

Prior to beginning your 5 X 5 Workout you will want to set a max of 5 repetitions for each exercise that you do and you want to make sure you don't go over 5 repetitions or under 5 repetitions.

You can warm-up by doing 5 easy repetitions of a light weight.

Then you want to slowly add weight as you begin your 5 X 5 workout by lifting weight that is challenging for you.

It is important to state that every time you go to the gym and exercise you will be adding 5 lbs. (pounds) to each of your exercises.

For example, if you bench press 135 pounds on Monday, then when you go back to the gym on Wednesday you will add 5 more pounds to your bench press so that you will now be bench pressing 140 pounds.

Once you find yourself having difficulty completing your 5 sets of 5 repetitions for all exercises after 3 days of nonconsecutive exercising, you then want to begin the deloading phase of the 5 X 5 Workout training program.

When you begin the deloading phase, you will subtract 10 pounds from your next workout.

For example, if on Monday you were struggling to bench press 5 sets of 5 repetitions at 140 pounds, then on Wednesday you would decrease the weight by removing 10 pounds from your bench press.

So now instead of trying to bench press 140 pounds you would instead bench press 130 pounds for your 5 X 5 Workout.

It is important to keep track of your workouts and how much you are lifting in order to know if you progressing and getting stronger.

Another variation of the 5 X 5 Workout is the Strong Lifts program.

So how does the Strong Lifts 5x5 program work?

For this program, you only work out **three days** a week using **two workout routines**. For example, look at the two workout routines below:

Workout Routine #1	Workout Routine #2
1. The Bench Press **(5 sets and 5 repetitions)** 2. The Squat **(5 sets and 5 repetitions)** 3. The Barbell Row **(5 sets and 5 repetitions)**	1. The Overhead Press **(5 sets and 5 repetitions)** 2. The Squat **(5 sets and 5 repetitions)** 3. The Deadlift **(1 set and 5 repetitions)**

So, on Monday you would do Workout Routine 1 then on Wednesday you would do Workout Routine 2.

Then, on Friday you would again do Workout Routine 1 again then you would rest on Saturday and Sunday.

You would repeat this cycle of alternating between workout routines throughout your training.

Here is another chart of how the training will take place throughout the week:

Monday	**Workout 1**
Tuesday	Rest
Wednesday	**Workout 2**
Thursday	Rest
Friday	**Workout 1**
Saturday	Rest
Sunday	Rest

It is important to state that for each lift, you perform 5 sets of 5 repetitions, with the exception of the deadlift, which is 1 set of 5 repetitions.

Although it may seem strange, according to the **Strong Lifts Program,** doing more exercise than what is recommended would cause undue stress to the body.

In addition, when you do compound exercises like the squat and deadlift, these exercises target a lot of muscles in the body.

Therefore, it is not recommended to do any additional exercises especially on consecutive days.

It is important to state that the Strong Lifts 5 X 5 Workout is not a bodybuilding program.

The goal of the Strong Lifts 5 X 5 Workout is to train in a somewhat small rep range in order to increase strength.

In addition, the Strong Lifts 5 X 5 Workout ensures that you increase the amount that you are lifting by 5 pounds each time you workout for as long as you can until you peak.

Some advantages of the Strong Lifts 5 X 5 Workout are:
1. It provides beginners with a base knowledge of an easy to follow strength training program.

2. The program only requires you to workout three days a week. So, you know how many days out of the week you need to train and exactly what exercises you should perform on your training days.

3. The program only requires you to focus on a few exercises instead of a wide variety of complex exercises.

4. The program also tells you exactly how many repetitions and sets you should perform for each exercise.

5. This program helps you to practice and master the exercises you perform in order to develop mastery with the program.

6. The program does not use machines. Instead the 5 X 5 Workout makes people get on their feet and teaches them to lift heavy.

It is important to state that although the Strong Lifts 5 X 5 Workout has many advantages, as with any workout program, there are also disadvantages as well.

For example, some intermediate and advanced strength training athletes believe the 5 X 5 training program is too simple.

To be more specific, some intermediate and advanced strength training athletes tend to need complexity and more variety in their training in order to continue to get stronger and remain motivated.

Some intermediate and advanced strength training athletes believe the 5 X 5 training program will only work for so long before they plateau and stop seeing improvements with their training.

Another disadvantage of the 5 X 5 Workout is that experienced lifters need to increase their training volume from 5 repetitions to as much as 15 repetitions in order to gain size and the 5 X 5 Workout does not recommend such high-volume training.

Last, if an experienced lifter is already strong it also does not offer adequate intensity to make him stronger.

There will also come a time when a lifter needs to lift very low reps for generating pure raw strength.

So, an experienced lifter may want to lift very low repetitions such as 3 reps, 2 reps, or even a 1 Rep Max and the 5 X 5 Workout simply does not recommend such low repetitions.

It is important to state that there is another variation of the 5 X 5 Workout called the Madcow 5 x 5 workout.

The Madcow 5 x 5 workout is recommended when the Strong Lifts 5x5 workout is no longer effective for your squat routine.

Something to consider with the 5 X 5 Workout is your age and body weight.

If you are say over 40 years old and have more than above body fat, it is recommended to switch from the Strong Lifts 5 X 5 Workout to the Madcow 5 X 5 Workout.

With the Madcow 5 X 5 Workout you will do the same workouts as you do in Strong Lifts with 3 modifications that will enhance your recovery from the progressively stressful workouts.

The Madcow 5 X 5 Workout will require you to do ramped up sets.

Ramped up sets are when you increase the weight you lift for every set by 5 lbs. (pounds).

In addition to doing the ramped up sets of 5 X 5 you will then complete the 5 X 5 workout with an intense 1 set x 5 repetitions.

For example, you will begin the Madcow 5 X 5 workout by bench pressing 135 lbs. (pounds) for 5 repetitions.

Your second set will be to bench press 140 lbs. (pounds) for 5 repetitions.

You will continue to add 5 lbs. (pounds) to your bench press until you reach the last set of the Madcow 5 X 5 workout.

On your last set you will do 1 set of 5 repetitions and this set will be your heaviest set.

Here is a chart that helps explain the Madcow 5 X 5 Workout:

Example of Madcow 5 X 5 Workout for Bench Press

1. Bench Press 135 lbs. X 5 repetitions
2. Bench Press 140 lbs. X 5 repetitions
3. Bench Press 145 lbs. X 5 repetitions
4. Bench Press 150 lbs. X 5 repetitions
5. Bench Press 155 lbs. X 5 repetitions *This will be your heaviest set

Unlike the Strong Lifts 5 x 5 Workout, the Madcow 5 X 5 Workout requires you to increase the weight you lift by 5 lbs. (pounds) every week instead of every time you work out like the Strong Lifts 5 x 5 Workout.

This is because at the intermediate level, the Madcow 5 X 5 Workout allows the body to have enough time to recover from every workout.

In addition, unlike the Strong Lifts 5 x 5 Workout, the Madcow 5 X 5 Workout also requires you to have 2 heavy squat days and 1 light squat day in a week instead of Strong Lift's recommended 3 heavy squat days in a week.

Here is a weekly schedule of how the Madcow 5 X 5 Workout looks:
(Monday) Workout 1:   Squat 1x5,   Bench Press 1x5, Barbell Rows 1x5
(Wednesday) Workout 2:   Squat 2x5,   Overhead Press 1x5, Deadlift 1x5
(Friday) Workout 3:   Squat 1x3,   Bench Press 1x3,   Barbell Rows 1x5
*Squat 1X5 means: 1 set of 5 Repetitions
*Squat 2X5 means: 2 sets of 5 repetitions
*Squat 1X3 means: 1 set of 3 reps

Keep in mind that the Madcow 5 X 5 Workout is a 5 set X 5 repetitions workout.

So, if the workout says you have to do Squats 2 X 5 this means that you first do 3 sets of 5 repetitions of squats followed by 2 sets of 5 repetitions of HEAVY squats (2X5).

Look at this example below:

Squat 2x5 (2 sets of 5 repetitions)

Ex) The first set is:	Squat 155 lbs. X 5 repetitions
The second set is:	Squat 160 lbs. X 5 repetitions
The third set is:	Squat 165 lbs. X 5 repetitions
The fourth set is:	Squat 170 lbs. X 5 repetitions
The fifth set is:	Squat 170 lbs. X 5 repetitions

So, as you can see from the example above both the fourth and the fifth sets will be the same weight which is what is meant by Squat 2 X 5.

Keep in mind that when you start the Madcow 5 X 5 Workout, you want to start lifting light rather than heavy.

While lifting light may be easy in the beginning you should focus on your technique and speed as you slowly increase the weight and progress to lifting more challenging weight.

Another variation of the 5 X 5 Workout is the Texas Method 5x5 workout.

The Texas Method 5x5 Workout is based on three strength training sessions a week.

In addition, you will be lifting 5 Rep Max (5RM) in four vital compound lifts which are the same as those from Strong Lifts.

To better understand what the 5 Rep Max (5RM) is, the 5 Rep Max (5RM) is basically lifting the heaviest weight that you can lift 5 times in a set.

In addition, the 5 Rep Max (5RM) should be approximately 85 percent of your 1 rep max.

For example, if your 1 rep max for the bench press is lifting 100 lbs. (pounds) then you would lift 85 percent of 100 lbs. (pounds) for 5 repetitions which is 5 repetitions of 85 lbs. (pounds) or 5 Rep Max (5RM).

Because you will be lifting approximately 85 percent of your 1 rep max with the Texas Method 5x5 Workout the goal is to rapidly increase your strength.

In addition, whenever you perform the Texas Method 5x5 Workout you need to make sure you use a "spotter," someone to help you, every time you workout.

You also want to make sure that you are not rushing your sets and are resting for adequate amounts of time between each set.

Here are some more tips for the Texas Method 5x5 Workout:

1. Maintain your schedule of having a rest day between your workouts.

2. Make sure you warm up before each exercise you perform.

3. Make sure to lift between 85-90 percent of your 5-rep max (5RM). Lifting 85-90 percent of your 5-rep max (5RM) will break down the maximum amount of muscle tissue needed to develop pure strength.

4. When doing your deadlifts, only do 1 set of 5 repetitions because they are a tough exercise and if you do more sets and repetitions, you will not be able to fully recover.

5. There are three workouts in the Texas Method 5x5 Workout and the second workout routine focuses on recovery.

6. The third workout routine is for intensity.

It is important to state that when it comes to gaining strength, you can choose to take a random approach and do random exercises for as long and hard as you can.

Or, you can follow a program like the 5 X 5 Workouts that are carefully and meticulously planned out to give you the best results possible.

In addition, the 5 X 5 Workouts include exercises that are manipulated over time for better intensity and volume.

Making sure you pick the right 5 X 5 Workout variation is crucial for better progress, fewer injuries, and making sure you push yourself as hard as you possibly can both night and day in order to achieve your strength training goals.

Chapter 4: Leg Exercises

The legs are the largest muscle group in the body.

When it comes to strength training, training the legs is extremely important because the legs along with your upper body will help you to develop a well-proportioned body.

Below are some very good leg exercises that you can include as part of your training.

Forward Lunges

Lunges are great leg exercise for developing strength, balance, coordination and conditioning.

Lunges can be performed using your bodyweight, dumbbells, barbells, medicine balls and so forth. In addition, there are also variations of the forward lunge.

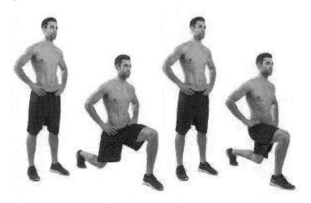

1. Start by setting your feet the width of your shoulders and place your arms on your hips.

2. Take a large step forward, keeping your back as straight as you can.

3. Lunge forward, making sure your front thigh is parallel with the ground and the back of your knee is as close to the floor as possible, but not quite reaching it.

4. You then step back coming back to the standing position and you will next lunge forward with the opposite let.

5. Do 3 sets of 10 to 15 reps per side.

6. To make the exercise more challenging you can dumbbells to lunge forward.

7. To make the exercise even more challenging you can use a barbell across your upper back to lunge forward.

   It is important to state that using a barbell across your upper back to lunge forward will truly work your core abdominal muscles because of the balance you will need to lunge forward with the bar laying across your upper back.

NOTE: When you lunge forward, both knees should be bent at 90-degree angles.

Backwards or Reverse Lunges

Reverse lunges are a great exercise that truly work your hamstrings and glutes.

In addition, the reverse lunge is less stressful on the knee than the forward lunge.

The reverse lunge may require a little more balance than the forward lunge. However, the reverse lunge is a powerful athletic strength training exercise.

The reverse lunge can be performed using your bodyweight, dumbbells, barbells, medicine balls and so forth. In addition, there are also variations of the reverse lunge.

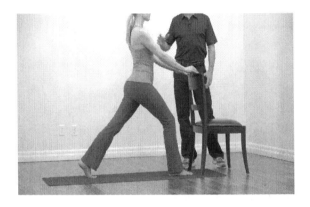

1. If you are a beginner to the reverse lunge you can use a chair to help you you're your balance.

   Using a chair, place your feet close to the back of the chair so that when you step back it prevents your knees from going past your toes.

   Execute a standing abdominal brace by pulling your belly button a little towards your spine. Keep your spine as upright as possible.

2. With your right leg, step back and position the ball of your foot on the floor.

   Keep your hips facing forward. This will inhibit your body from twisting.

   Keep your spine straight and bend both knees to lower your body down. <u>Only use the back of the chair for support if you need it.</u>

3. Push into the floor with your left leg as you rise to the standing position. Repeat this movement for 10-15 repetitions and then switch sides. To achieve maximum benefits, your movements should be slow and steady.

   Note: Using a barbell across your upper back for a reverse lunge will truly work your core abdominal muscles because of the balance you will need to lunge backwards with the bar laying across your upper back.

Olympic Lifts

Olympic exercises have become very popular in the past few years as a result of their powerful benefits.

Olympic lifts are great for developing strength, speed, power, coordination, conditioning and flexibility.

Some Olympic lifts consists of the Snatch and the Power Clean.

These powerful exercises take tremendous dedication and proper technique in order to master.

You will need to ensure you give these exercises your complete concentration on your body position and technique.

You should only focus on practicing one Olympic lift at a time and make sure to master that specific Olympic lift.

After you feel you have mastered a specific Olympic lift it is time to move on and master another Olympic lift.

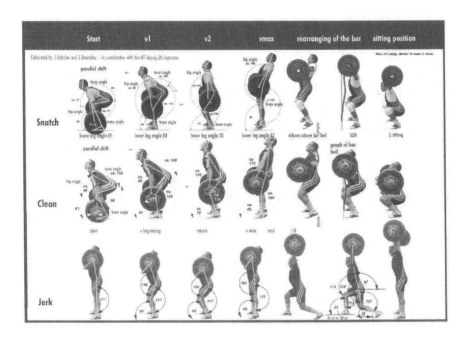

The Leg Press

The Leg Press is a good exercise to use for a lower body workout.

Although some people may think that the leg press is an exercise for beginners, many advanced lifters can also benefit from the leg press.

The leg press can be used to build strength.

In addition, the leg press can be a good exercise to build functional strength especially when you do the one-legged press.

The leg press can also be an alternative to squats when you simply feel a little too tired from your previous squat session.

In addition, the leg press machine can even be used to exercise your calf muscles.

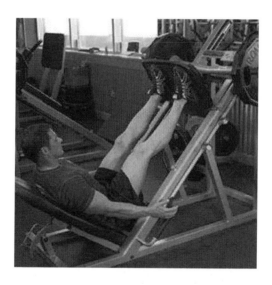

To learn how to use the Leg Press machine begin by sitting on the machine and put your legs in front of you with your feet the same width as your shoulders.

Gradually lower the safety bars holding the weighted platform in place and press the platform all the way up until your legs are completely extended in front of you.

Note: **Ensure that you do not lock your knees.** Your torso and the legs should make a perfect 90-degree angle. This is your starting position.

As you breathe in, gradually lower the platform until your lower and upper legs make a 90-degree angle.

Use your quadriceps and legs to go back and forth pushing the weight.

Make sure to breathe in and out as you perform this exercise and make sure to push with the heels of your feet as you perform this exercise.

Perform 10-15 repetitions and make sure you lock the safety pins properly once you are done with the exercise.

Additional Leg Exercises

Barbell Squats

Barbell squats are considered the king of leg exercises.

This is one exercise you really want to make sure you focus on your technique and your breathing.

It is recommended to do between 10-15 repetitions of barbell squats for maximum strength.

However, there is also a 20-rep barbell squat challenge that you can consider doing.

Note: the 20-rep barbell squat challenge is very difficult to do.

You instead want to begin by slowly increasing your squat repetitions in a span of a few months in order to develop the stamina required to undertake the 20-rep squat challenge.

Dumbbell squats

Dumbbell squats are a great exercise for developing your legs. Dumbbell squats can be used when a squat rack may not be available.

Jumping squats

Jumping squats are great for developing strength, speed and power. In the beginning, you can use your own bodyweight and as you progress you can begin to use light dumbbells.

Jumping squats can be exhausting because your body uses so much energy to push you off the ground.

Try to do between 5-10 repetitions and slowly progress with using light dumbbells to better challenge yourself.

Bodyweight Squats

Bodyweight squats are great for beginners. In addition, bodyweight squats can be used as a good warmup before doing barbell squats.

Bodyweight squats can also help you to practice your technique for barbell squats. Once you have mastered the bodyweight squat, it is time to move on to either dumbbell squats or the more challenging barbell squats.

Barbell step-ups

Barbell step-ups are great for developing strength for each length individually.

Barbell step-ups can be challenging because for a brief moment you will be lifting weight using only one leg.

However, you will develop balance, coordination and strength with barbell step-ups and you will become more functional as a result of practicing barbell step-ups.

In the beginning you can use your own bodyweight in order to learn the mechanics of properly doing step-ups.

Once you are comfortable doing bodyweight step-ups, you can progress to dumbbell step-ups.

A word of caution, dumbbell step-ups can quickly fatigue the hands and forearms so it is a good idea to use light to moderate weight when performing the dumbbell step-up.

After you have gone through the process of mastering the bodyweight and dumbbell step-up, you can then move on to the more challenging barbell step-up.

Chapter 5: Back Exercises

The back muscles are the second largest group of muscles in the body. In addition, the back muscles are made of so many muscles.

Therefore, it is important to do various exercises for your back.

Here are some good exercises for training you back:

Deadlift: muscles worked- legs and upper back

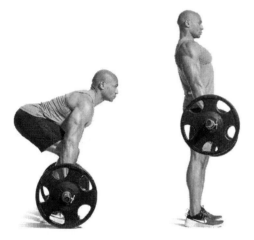

1. Begin by walking towards the bar, standing with the middle of your foot positioned under the bar. Do not have your shins touch the bar. Your feet should be hip-width apart with your toes pointed out 15 degrees.

2. Grasp the bar with your hands placed approximately the width of your shoulders and your arms should be vertical from the front view and hanging right outside your legs.

3. Your knees should be bent until your shins touch the bar. Do not move the bar. Keep it over the middle of your foot.

4. Elevate your chest and keep your back straight. Do not move the bar or have your hips drop. Also, do not squeeze your shoulder blades.

5. Pull. Inhale deeply, holding it while you stand up. Keep the bar against your legs. Don't shrug or lean back at the top.

Bent-Over Barbell Rows

Bent over barbell rows are an excelling total body exercise. The barbell row works your arms, back, lower back and legs. The more parallel you are to the floor the more challenging the exercise becomes.

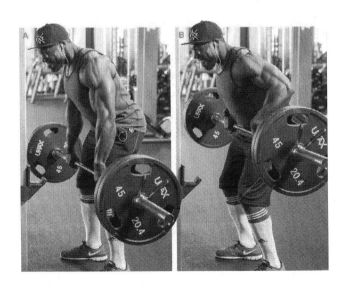

Instructions for the Bent over Barbell Row

Hold the barbell with your palms facing down, bending your knees somewhat and bring your torso frontward, by bending at the waist, while you keep the back straight until it is nearly parallel to the floor.

Note: Ensure that you keep your head up. The barbell should hang straight in front of you as your arms hang perpendicular to your torso and the floor. This will be your starting position.

Now, keep your torso still, exhale and lift the barbell towards you.

Keep your elbows close to your body and only use your forearms to hold the weight.

At the top constricted position, squeeze your back muscles and hold it there for a brief pause.

Then breathe in and gently lower the barbell back to the starting position. Repeat for the desired amount of repetitions.

Additional Back Exercises

Wide grip pull-ups

Wide grip pull-ups are an excellent challenging exercise that will work not only your back muscles but also your entire upper body.

More specifically, you will be working your lats (back muscles), your shoulders, your chest, your biceps, your torso and your forearms with wide grip pullups.

Before you begin doing wide grip pull-ups, you want to warm-up by doing close grip pull-ups and then slowly progress to wide grip pull-ups.

It is important to state that wide grip pull-ups can put some strain on the front shoulder.

As a result, make sure you properly warm-up by doing close grip pull-ups and then slowly widen your grip and perform wide grip pull-ups.

One Arm Dumbbell Rows

One arm dumbbell rows are great for isolating the back muscles and allowing you to build strength in the back muscles.

You can even do what's called "drop sets" with one arm dumbbell rows which will challenge you even more.

Close grip T-bar Rows

Close grip T-bar rows are like barbell bent over rows except that T-bar rows require you to have a very close grip.

Close grip T-bar rows are great for building a strong back.

Dumbbell Pull-Over

The dumbbell pull-over is a great upper body exercise.

This exercise not only works your back muscles but it also works your chest muscles as well.

Famous bodybuilder Arnold Schwarzenegger was such a big advocate of the dumbbell pull-over that he would do it at the end of every workout.

Chapter 6: Chest Exercises

The chest is the third largest muscle group in the body. Believe it or not but when you do exercises like the squat and wide grip pull-ups you are also exercising your chest muscles.

Here are some great chest exercises that you can apply to your training:

Top Chest Building Exercises

1. Dumbbell Close Grip Squeeze Press

The close grip dumbbell press is an exercise that will target the center of your chest as well as your triceps.

It is important to state that you can also perform this exercise using a barbell.

In addition, you can also do variations of the dumbbell bench press using an incline and decline bench.

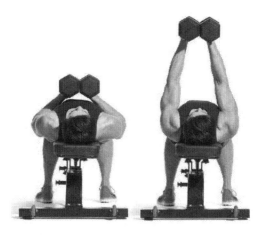

a. Lie down on a bench and hold a pair of dumbbells with your arms above your chest, palms facing each other.

Allow the weights to touch and squeeze them together as hard as you can.

Maintaining the squeeze, make sure the dumbbells stay in contact with each other.

Lower the dumbbells to the sides of your chest.

Next, push the dumbbells upwards, back to the beginning position.

2. Barbell Flat Bench Press

The barbell bench press is a great upper body exercise.

The barbell bench press works your chest, abs, and arms.

Perform the barbell bench press at the beginning of your chest workout.

For a more complete chest workout vary the grip width. Also, make sure to warm-up using light weights before performing the barbell bench press.

It is important to state that you can also do variations of the barbell bench press using an incline and decline bench.

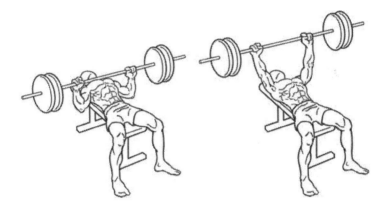

a. Begin the barbell bench press by sitting at the end of your bench and then lie down by lowering yourself back on the bench. Place your eyes underneath the bar.

b. Elevate your chest and tense your upper back. Place your shoulder blades down and back and then squeeze them.

c. Place your pinky finger on the inside of the rings. Hold the bar low and close to your wrist. Clasp the bar using the complete grip to prevent it from moving.

d. Set your feet flat on the floor in a stance that is approximately the width of your shoulders. One at a time, set your feet underneath your knees.

e. To lift the bar out of the rack, straighten your arms.

f. Lift or bench press the barbell for 8-12 reps and do between 4-6 sets including 2 warm-up sets.

g. Make sure to warm-up properly before you begin to lift heavy.

3. **Flat Bench Dumbbell Bench Press**

The dumbbell bench press is an excellent alternative to the barbell bench press.

The dumbbell bench press can be considered to be a better chest exercise than the barbell bench press because the dumbbell bench press allows for more range of motion on the descending part of the exercise.

In addition, the dumbbell bench press corrects imbalances with the chest and arms as a result of each arm working individually to push the weight up and down.

It is important to state that you can also do variations of the dumbbell bench press using an incline and decline bench.

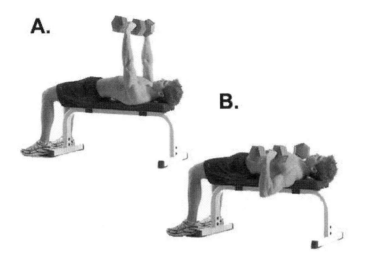

Just like the barbell bench press, the dumbbell bench press should be done at the beginning of your exercise routine.

4. Incline Bench Cable Fly

The incline cable fly is an excellent exercise that works the upper chest.

One thing to mention about the incline cable fly is that you have to make sure your arms stretch out parallel to the floor and do not go past parallel.

In addition, the cable fly places a lot of stress on the front shoulder so you have to make sure you monitor the weight and have excellent technique when performing this exercise.

Some variations of the incline cable fly are:
- Standing cable flys
- Dumbbells flys
- Flat bench flys

- Decline bench flys

Note: Do this exercise towards the end of your chest routine.

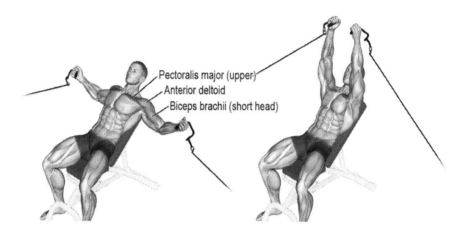

a. You should start with your hands to your sides with your elbows slightly bent.

b. Place an incline bench in the middle of two cable stacks in a cable crossover machine.

c. You need to set the cable pulleys to the lowest position and lie back on the bench. Next, you will take hold of the cable handles.

d. Begin with your hands straight out to the sides. They should be approximately shoulder height. Do not lock your elbows. They should be slightly bent.

e. As you contract your chest muscles, you will pull your hands up and together until the handles are almost touching. You should be maintaining the same bent elbow position throughout the exercise. Do not lock them or bend them further.

f. Your finishing position will be with your hands together directly above your chest. Once you are in the top position, you will want to contract your chest muscles a little more to maximize the contraction.

g. Do 3 or 4 sets consisting of 10 to 12 repetitions per set.

5. Incline Dumbbell Pull-Over

The incline dumbbell pull-over is a great upper body exercise that works the upper muscles of the chest.

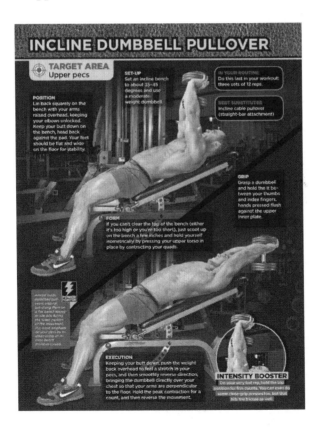

a. Lie on the bench so that only your shoulders are being supported.

b. Keep your feet flat on the floor, approximately the width of your shoulders.

c. Your head and neck will be hanging over the bench.

d. Your hips should be preferably at a somewhat lower angle than your shoulders

e. Hold the dumbbell with your hands positioned in a diamond (rhombus) shape using your thumbs and fingers. Your palms need to be facing the ceiling.

f. The movement will start with the dumbbell over your chest and your elbows should be bent 10 to15 degrees. Do not change this at any point throughout the exercise.

g. Take a deep breath and inhale deeply and hold it while you slowly lower the weight backward over your head until your upper arms are aligned with your torso. Your arms should be parallel to the floor.

h. The weight will travel in an arc-like motion towards the floor.

i. Breathe out and pull the dumbbell back so that it is directly over your chest again, purposely squeezing your chest muscles.

j. Hold for a brief second, and then repeat the exercise for between 8-12 repetitions.

6. Incline Dumbbell Bench Press

The incline dumbbell bench press is an excellent chest exercise.

The incline dumbbell bench press targets the upper chest muscles and shoulders more than the flat bench dumbbell press.

The incline dumbbell bench press is definitely more challenging than the flat dumbbell bench press.

As a result, you will lift less weight than the flat bench dumbbell press.

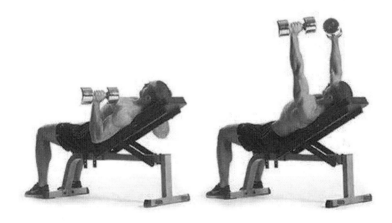

a. Set the bench backrest to a 45-degree angle.

Hold a pair of dumbbells with your arms above your chest with your palms facing your feet.

Bring the dumbbells down to your chest level and then raise (press) them back up to the beginning position.

7. Incline Barbell Bench Press

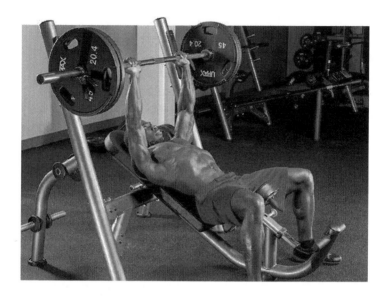

a. The incline barbell press should also be the primary exercise in chest training for bodybuilders and anyone that wants to develop strength.

The Incline barbell press is an extremely popular exercise with the bodybuilding and strength training community. So, do the incline barbell press in addition to the flat bar bench press for building the chest muscles.

Incline Barbell Bench Press - How it's done:

A. On an incline bench, lean back at approximately 30 to 45 degrees. Your feet need to be flat on the floor in order to give yourself a good, sturdy base.

Your lower back should be flat against the bench. Slightly arch your back during this lift.

Grab the bar with a wide or medium grip. When you get the bar off of the rack, do not go down instantly with it.

Raise the bar off of the rack and hold it for a second or two right above your head with your arms locked. This will help you to get oriented with it first.

B. Begin going down with the weight gradually until you touch the muscles of the upper chest near the bottom of the chin.

Pause for a moment so that you do not bounce the weight off your chest, then raise the weight back up to the top position, breathing out on the way back up. Keep in mind, if you touch the nipple area, you went too low.

C. The bar should be positioned so that it either touches your chin or just below your chin. Going even an inch too low takes the emphasis off the objective area.

You need to keep your wrists straight and your elbows below your wrists with your arms placed at a 45 degree angle.

Do not keep your elbows back because this puts maximum a lot of stress on the chest muscles and places severe stress on the shoulder joint.

*Perform between 8-12 repetitions.

8. Weighted Pushups

Weighted pushups are a great bodyweight exercise that work your chest, arms, abs and shoulders.

You can challenge yourself by placing a 10, 25, 35 or even 45 lb. (pound) plate on your back.

Research shows that the weighted pushup is the equivalent of doing the heavy barbell bench press.

How to do the Weighted Pushup

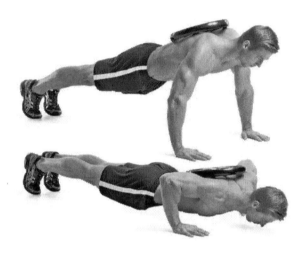

a. Kneel down like if you are going to get into a pushup position. Next grab a barbell plate and carefully place it on your upper back.

   Note: The weighted push-up can also be performed wearing a weighted vest.

   Your arms should be straight and hands should be placed a little wider apart than your shoulders.

   Bend at the elbows and lower your body until your chest almost touches the floor. Pause and then push your body back up.

9. Close Grip Bench Press

The close grip bench press is a chest exercise that heavily targets the triceps muscles.

Because the triceps are heavily targeted, you will not be able to bench press very heavy weight.

However, you will be working the center of your chest and your triceps and this makes for a good chest exercise.

Note: Your wrists may become sore as a result of the hand positioning with this exercise.

How to Do the Close Grip Bench Press

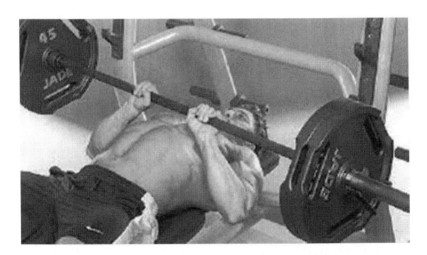

   a.   Begin by using an overhand grip that is a little narrower than the width of your shoulders and hold the barbell above the sternum with your arms straightened.

        Lower the bar to your chest and hold for 1 second. Press the bar back up to the starting position.

Do between 8-12 repetitions.

10. Chest Squeeze Pushup

The chest squeeze pushup is like the close grip bench press except that you use dumbbells and the position is similar to that of doing a pushup.

The chest squeeze pushup will work the center of the chest as well as the triceps.

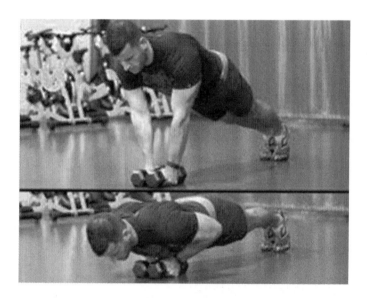

How to Do the Chest Squeeze Pushup

a. Begin by placing two dumbbells next to each other. You want to make sure they are touching and the handles are parallel to each other. Next, get into the standard push-up position.

STRENGTH TRAINING (SECRETS)

b. Grab a dumbbell with each hand. Keep your arms straight and your body should form a straight line, from ankles to head. Press the weights together forcefully. Lower your body until your chest almost touches the floor.

c. Push your body back up to the starting position, ensuring that you do not stop squeezing the dumbbells together.

Do between 8-12 reps for maximum strength.

If you want to challenge yourself even more, place a 10 or 25 lb. (pound) plate on your back and perform "close grip weighted pushups."

Barbells vs Dumbbells – Which is Better???

Dumbbells - Here are some reasons why dumbbells are better than barbells:

1. Dumbbells can be safer than barbells especially for beginners.
2. Dumbbells allow for more range of motion (ROM) when compared to barbells.
3. Dumbbells can correct muscle imbalances.
4. Dumbbells have a more free "natural" feel of moving and lifting weights than barbells do.
5. Dumbbells can help you develop strength evenly throughout your body.
6. Dumbbells make great use of the stabilizer muscles.
7. Dumbbells can sometimes be easier to use than barbells.

Barbells - Here are some reasons why barbells are better than dumbbells:

1. Barbells allow you to lift heavier weight than dumbbells.
2. Barbells will not fatigue your hands and forearms the way dumbbells do especially for exercises like the dumbbell lunge.
3. Barbells allow you to generate more power for explosive Olympic exercises than dumbbells.
4. Barbells can be easier to use than dumbbells when it comes to lifting very heavy weights especially for exercises like squats and deadlifts.
5. Barbells can be more practical than dumbbells when it comes to exercises like the deadlift.

The Verdict – So which is Better Dumbbells or Barbells???

Both dumbbells and barbells are essential when it comes to strength training and building the body you want.

You have to experiment with using both dumbbells and barbells and figure out what works best for you.

In addition, using both dumbbells and barbells as part of your training will help you to develop both strength and correct any muscular imbalances you may have in your body.

As a result, don't limit yourself to only a handful of exercises or pieces of equipment.

Instead, look at strength training and building the body you desire with an open mind and if you do so, you will most certainly achieve your fitness goals.

Chapter 7: Mastering the Barbell Squat with Proper Form

How to enhance your butt muscles

There are three muscles that make up the butt: **the gluteus maximus (G-max), gluteus medius (G-med), and gluteus minimus (G-min).**

The primary muscle is the gluteus maximus (G-max) and it is the largest muscle in the body.

The function of the gluteus maximus (G-max) is for movement of the leg specifically the thigh and hip.

The functions of the gluteus medius (G-med) and gluteus minimus (G-min) are quite similar.

They move toward the thigh, stabilize the leg during the single support phase of running and internally (with a flexed hip) and externally (with an extended hip) rotate the thigh.

It is important to state that barbell squats have the potential to make your butt bigger through constant stimulation.

In addition, working the glute muscles will give you a better chance of sculpting your butt.

Contrary to popular belief, constantly clenching your butt also known as **perma-clenching** is not good for you.

Perma-clenching leads to increased wear on your lumbar discs and sacroiliac joints.

In addition, perma-clenching decreases core support, causes hip pain and causes the pelvic to be too tight.

Barbell Squats - The Total Body Workout

Squats create total body strength, improve athleticism, and stimulate total body muscle growth.

This is why squats are considered royalty in the lifting world.

The only problem is many people do not have enough mobility or ability to squat not only safely, but effectively as well.

It is important to state that you need mobility to achieve proper form and stability to control your movements through squats intended range of motion.

The 5 Mistakes People Make with the Squat

1. The first mistake many people make when squatting is not stretching or performing mobility work before they begin squatting.

   Stretching and performing mobility work should be done throughout the week in order to increase flexibility throughout the legs, hips and thighs.

   In addition to not stretching or performing mobility work before squatting, if your shoulders are tight, chances are when you use a barbell during your squat routine, all the weight ends up being pressed onto your neck and you run the risk of compressing spinal disks and pinching nerves.

This could lead to a multitude of other problems such as pain on your neck, back, knees, and even your feet.

To counteract and prevent this from happening, perform shoulder warm-up exercises to increase mobility and prevent injuries.

For tight hips, perform some slow and controlled leg swings, do some light jogging and even some basic bodyweight squats will loosen up your hips.

2. The second mistake many people make when squatting is stopping at 90 degrees.

   To build muscle when squatting, you need to go as low as possible for every repetition.

   The lower you squat, the more you activate your glutes and hamstrings.

   Powerlifting stops just below 90 degrees when it comes to squatting. In addition, bodybuilding requires squatting all the way down, known as Ass to Grass (ATG).

   When performing Ass to Grass Squats you want to make sure that the barbell is placed on your upper back and that the weight of the barbell is directly above your hips for proper positioning.

3. The third mistake many people make when squatting is pressing from their toes.

As you squat low and are getting ready to stand you want to make sure that you are pressing from the heels and through the middle of your feet and NOT your toes to finish your reps.

You should be bending at your knees and hips at the same time as you go down.

Then come back up to a standing position and push strongly from the heels all the way through the middle of your foot.

As you squat down, you want to make sure that your heels don't come off the ground, because by doing so you will be putting tremendous pressure on your toes which puts a lot of stress on your knees.

This pressure and on your toes can lead to foot and knee injuries.

In order to master the barbell squat, you want to make sure that you practice the exercise in a fluid movement without any weight until you master proper positioning.

Keep in mind that if your knees bend inward while squatting, you need to stop immediately to correct your form.

Bending of the knees inward can cause ACL tears.

To correct this, you can widen your stance or slightly point your toes outward.

Widening your stance will prevent your knees from bending inward.

4. The fourth mistake people make when performing barbell squats is they do not breathe during their repetitions and instead hold their breath.

Holding your breath while squatting can make you dizzy and cause you to lose core stability as well as cause you to faint and collapse.

When performing barbell squats, you want to make sure that you keep your core nice and strong and you also want to make sure that you ALWAYS keep proper form.

To do this, make sure you practice taking deep breaths as well as keeping your core tight and flexing your abdominal muscles.

In addition, make sure you exhale as you perform barbell squats and always be aware of your breathing when performing this tough exercise.

5. The fifth mistake people make when performing barbell squats is not resting enough in between sets.

In order to ensure quality reps, you need to rest 2-3 minutes in between sets in order to allow your body adequate recovery time.

This is especially true when performing high repetition barbell squats such as sets of 15 repetitions or more.

When performing barbell squats for low repetitions such as 3-5 repetitions, you should rest 3-5 minutes in between sets.

It is important to state that resting too long can "cool down" the body which will prevent you from performing at your maximum performance as well as lead to injury.

The 10 Best Ways to Boost Your Squat Routine

1. **Train for Maximum Strength.** You need to develop a base of absolute strength.

2. **Train for Power with Submaximal Repetitions.** So simply train with strength and speed. Training for power can be achieved with speed squats.

3. **Train for speed, strength and power.** Jump squats are good for this.

4. **Squat twice a week.** For full recovery, allow 48-72 hours between barbell squat sessions.

5. **Train for Squat Depth.** If you cannot maintain proper form because of a lack of core control, do not force a deep squat.

    In addition, if you lack flexibility around your hips and thighs, then you need to improve on your flexibility and mobility before doing Ass To Grass (ATG) Squats.

6. **Do not forget about your front squats.** The benefits of **front squats** include similar muscle activation as the back squat without as much joint compression and stress as a result of squatting less weight.

In addition, when performing front squats your core muscles will be working very hard to make sure you have proper form when executing this tough exercise.

It is important to mention that front squats will be working more of your quad muscles as a result of all the weight being placed at the front of the body.

7. **Widen your stance.** You want to make sure you point your toes a little outward as well as your knees during barbell squats in order to prevent your knees from collapsing or bending inward.

Having a wide stance while performing barbell squats will emphasize hip and posterior chain development and increase your squat repetitions.

8. **Train in various rep ranges.** Practice doing high repetitious for strength endurance as well as low repetitions for pure strength.

9. **Bend the Bar.** Engage the lats, create additional stability in the trunk, and have full control of the heavy barbell by driving your elbows down and back.

You will also prevent the bar from jumping off your back during explosive squats if you have complete control of the heavy barbell.

Note: It may be safer to use dumbbells for explosive or jumping squats.

10. **Rack at the Correct Height.** The squat rack should be set up with the barbell set in the middle of the nipple and shoulder height.

This is low enough to permit you to squat and rack the weight safely.

Squatting with Proper Form

1. Squat with your heels shoulder-width apart as well as with your heels under your shoulders.

2. Turn your feet out 30 degrees, keeping your whole foot flat on the floor. Don't raise your toes or heels while squatting.

3. Drive your knees to the side, in the direction of your feet, locking your knees at the top of each rep.

4. Bend your knees and hips at the same time. Shift your hips back and down while thrusting your knees out.

5. Bend with a natural arch in your lower back like when you stand. No rounding or extra arching while squatting. Keep your back in a neutral position.

6. Squeeze the barbell fiercely but do not try to maintain heavy weight with your hands. Let your upper back support the barbell.

7. Use an average grip, thinner than when you Bench Press. Your hands should be further than the width of your shoulders.

8. Place the bar in between your traps and rear shoulders also known as a low bar, or on your traps also known as the high bar. Then center the bar on your upper back.

9. Your wrists will hurt and bend if you try to brace the bar with your hands. Support the weight of the barbell with your upper-back.

10. Elbows should be at the back of your torso at the very top before you squat. Make sure to keep your back straight and upright at the bottom of the squat.

11. Curve the upper portion of your back to establish support for the bar. Compress your shoulder blades and inflate your chest.

12. Elevate your chest before you un-rack the bar. Keep it raised and firm by inhaling deeply before you Squat down.

13. Keep your head aligned with your torso. Do not look at the ceiling or your feet. Also, do not turn your head to the right or left.

14. Your back angle should always be diagonal, not vertical or horizontal. The precise back angle depends on your body type and the bar position.

15. Place the bar on your back and put your feet under the bar. Remove the barbell from the rack by straightening your legs. Slowly walk back before you squat.

16. On the way down, bend your hips and knees simultaneously. Hips should be back with the knees out, keeping your lower back neutral.

17. Squat down until your hips are below your knees. If your thighs are parallel to the floor, you are not squatting far enough.

18. Move your hips upright, keeping your knees out, your chest elevated and your head neutral.

19. Between reps, stand with your hips and knees locked straight. Inhale and exhale while you get ready for the next repetition.

20. Lock your knees and hips. Step forward toward the squat rack. Then bend your knees to place the barbell on the squat rack.

21. Transport the bar in a vertical line above the middle of your foot. Do not perform any horizontal movements.

22. At the top, take in a deep breath and hold it at the bottom. Breathe out at the top.

The Active Squat/ Chair Pose

The active squat/chair pose is good for practicing mobility and flexibility as well as for warming up the body before doing barbell squats.

In addition, the active squat/chair pose is also good for learning the mechanics of how to squat properly before moving on to doing barbell squats.

The active squat/chair pose is also great for decreasing lower back tension, as well as preventing fatigue from sitting for extended periods of time and for eliminating tightness around the hips.

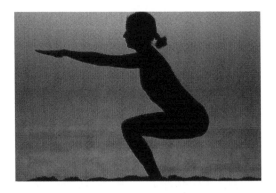

How to Do the Active Squat/ Chair Pose

1. First stand firmly

2. Next, bend your knees and slowly get into the proper squat position.

3. You then want to contract your Gluteus Maximus (G-max), adductor magnus and your hamstrings while holding the squat position for 30 seconds.

4. Make, sure to contract all three at the same time while holding the squat position for 30 seconds.

***If you begin to experience any knee pain while practicing the active squat/chair pose simply do the following:

1. Only bend your knees a couple of degrees and don't squat so low.

2. Widen or narrow your feet position based on your comfort level.

3. Use a wall and lean against it to practice the squat/chair pose.

Chapter 8: Recipes

Drinks #1

Bounce Back Smoothie

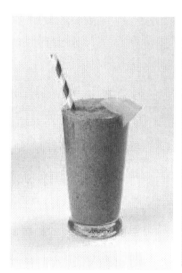

Nutrition Facts	
Number of Servings: 2	
Amount Per Serving	
Calories 227	
Protein 20g	
Carbs 30g	
Fat 3g	
Fiber 6g	

Notice: Eating the right diet for your goals may result in increased gains and decreased bodyfat.

- Prep time takes about 5 minutes
- Cook time takes about a minute
- This serves 2 people

What's in it:
- 1 cup of Almond Milk
- ½ cup of Blueberries
- 1 tablespoon of Honey
- 1 medium Banana
- 1 cup of Spinach

- 2 tablespoons of Greek Yogurt
- 3 medium sized Strawberries
- 1 scoop of Protein Powder

Instructions:
1. Put all ingredients together in a blender.
2. Blend for 30 seconds.
3. Drink

Drinks #2

Lean and Green Meal Replacement Smoothie

What's in it:
- 1/4 cup of Water
- 1/4 cup of Pineapple
- 1 scoop of Lean Body Natural Protein
- 1/4 oz. of Wheatgrass
- 3 Strawberries (raw or freshly frozen)
- 1/3 of a Banana
- 1/2 of Small Avocado
- 1 cup of Chopped Kale
- Add ice for thickness

Instructions for Lean and Green Meal Replacement Smoothie

1. Put all ingredients into a blender and blend for about 1 minute.

2. You can freeze the fruit to chill the smoothie rather than using ice.

3. If you would like to add more complex carbs and make a thicker shake and make it more filling, add 1/4 cup of uncooked oatmeal.

4. When ready, drink.

Meals

Meal #1
Breakfast

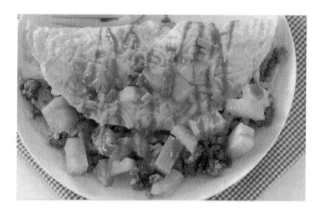

High Protein Cheese and Beef Omelet

- Prep takes about 15 minutes
- Cook Time takes about 10 minutes
- This serves 1 person

What's in it?

- 2 large Eggs
- Salt & Pepper, as desired
- 1/4 cup of Egg Whites

- Ketchup
- 2 tablespoons of Reduced Fat Cheddar Cheese
- Sliced Pickles
- 1/4 cup of Sliced Tomatoes
- Any other toppings you wish to add
- 4 oz. Lean Ground Beef

Nutrition Facts

Amount Per Serving

Calories 409

Protein 50g

Carbs 12g

Fat 16g

Notice: Eating the right diet for your goals may result in increased gains and decreased bodyfat.

Cooking Instructions:

1. Mix eggs.

2. Over medium heat, heat up skillet. Then add eggs onto skillet.

3. Cook eggs until desired. Remove from heat.

4. Cook ground beef, salt, and pepper in a second skillet. When done, spread the ground beef over one side of the cooked eggs.

5. Top with tomato and pickles.

6. Fold eggs over beef.

7. Sprinkle cheese on top.

8. Cover and cook on low until cheese is somewhat melted.

Note: For a vegetarian-friendly dish, replace beef with tofu and cheese with soy crumbles.

Meal #2

<u>Banana, Blueberry and Oatmeal Pancakes</u>

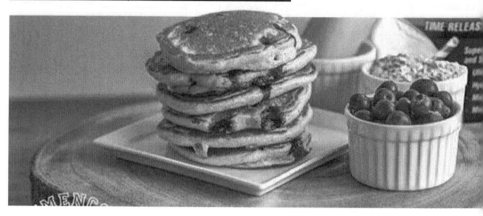

What's in it?

- 2 tablespoons of baking powder
- 1/2 cup of blueberries
- 1/2 medium banana
- 1/2 cup of oatmeal, uncooked
- 1/2 cup of egg whites (or 3 egg whites)
- 1 scoop whey protein
- 1 or 2 cups of milk or water

Cooking Instructions:
1. Put oatmeal in blender or food processor.

2. Add 1 or 2 cups of milk or water to the blender.

3. Add eggs, baking powder, banana, and scoop of whey protein. Blend on pulse until smooth.

4. Put blueberries in the mix and stir with a spatula or spoon.

5. Put skillet on med-high heat and measure approximately 2 tablespoons of batter per pancake.

6. Cover pancakes with a lid while they cook to help the inside cook faster. Cook them for approximately 45 seconds to 1 minute on the first side, and then approximately 30 seconds to 45 seconds on the other side.

Nutrition Facts
Calories: 544
Fat: 11 g
Carbs: 64
Protein: 47 g

Meal #3 Dinner

Lean Beef Spinach Meatball Pasta

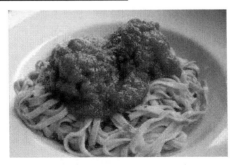

Prep time takes between 5 and 10 minutes
Cook time takes about 10 to 12 minutes

This serves 1 person

What's needed for the meatballs?
- Sea salt and pepper, for taste
- 1/2 tablespoon of cumin
- 1 tablespoon of garlic, minced
- 1/4 cup of diced red onion
- 1/2 cup of shredded raw spinach
- 6 oz. of lean ground beef

Ingredients for pasta:

- 2 oz of wheat spinach pasta
- 1 tablespoon of low-fat parmesan cheese
- 5 cherry tomatoes
- 1 and 1/2 cup of raw spinach
- 1 tablespoon of marinara (natural, low sodium)

Instructions:
1. Preheat the oven to 400 degrees Fahrenheit.

2. Sauté red onions in skillet (for flavor) using coconut or olive oil.

3. Mix together the ground beef, red onion, shredded spinach, minced garlic, and spices.

4. Shape one or two meatballs approximately the size of your hands. Use a food scale if you would like them to be proportionate.

5. Set the meatballs on a baking sheet and place them in a preheated oven. Cook for 10 to 12 minutes.

6. Cook pasta. When the pasta is done cooking, mix in spinach, cheese, and tomatoes, as desired.

Nutrition Facts
Calories: 468
Fat: 6 g
Carbs: 50 g
Protein: 51 g

Snacks/ Desserts

Banana Split with Protein Ice Cream

What's in it?
- 1 medium-large sized banana
- 1 cup of vanilla ice-cream
- 7 oz of Greek yogurt
- 1/2 cup of whey protein
- Optional: 3 diced/ chopped strawberries

Nutrition Facts
Calories: 493
Fat: 12 g
Carbs: 49 g
Protein: 47 g

Instructions:

1. Mix Greek yogurt, whey protein and vanilla ice-cream in a bowl. Mix until smooth.

2. Put bowl in refrigerator for 1.5 to 2 hours or until it is your desired firmness.

3. Slice banana vertically in half and place in separate bowl.

4. Remove ice cream from freezer. Dig out the ice cream with an ice cream scoop and place on top of banana.

5. Add fresh fruit, if desired.

NOTE: To increase the protein content, simply add 1 full scoop of whey protein. To add more carbs, use one whole banana.

Chapter 9: Short Glossary

1RM: "One Repetition Max"; the maximum amount of weight that you can lift for a given exercise.

Heavy Lifting: 85 percent (or more) of your maximum effort for multiple sets of 1-5 repetitions

Hypertrophy: Excessive development of an organ or part of the body.

Hypertrophy training is particularly used to increase in bulk (as by the thickening of muscle fibers). You basically gain size when doing hypertrophy training.

Periodization: Changing a strength training program as you advance through the workout by challenging your muscles further each week and then having enough recovery time built in with an easier week so you do not become overtrained.

Perma-clenching: clenching your butt constantly.

Traps: Short for trapezius. The traps are large muscles that run along the back side of your neck and along your spine.

Its functions are to move the scapulae and support the arm.

Conclusion

Thanks for making it through to the end of this book.

I hope it was informative and able to provide you with all of the tools you need to achieve your strength training goals.

The next step is to start implementing what you learned into your strength training routine.

Make sure you are getting an adequate amount of rest as it is not only beneficial to your body and mind but it also affects your strength training regimen.

You now know the basics of strength training and how to get started if you have never done anything like it before.

This will then lead you into the 5x5 workout and some of the best workouts for your legs, chest, and back.

Keep in mind that it is important to pick the exercises that are right for you.

You have also learned about the **"King Exercise of Strength Training: The Barbell Squat."**

In addition, you have learned some recipes that are ideal for all your nutritional needs so that you can come up with meal plans that are suitable for your training needs.

Take it upon yourself to learn as much as you can about strength training through trial and error.

In addition, experiment with various strength training programs, routines and workouts so that you can always be evolving and never plateau with your strength training goals.

You have learned what is needed in order for you to achieve your strength training goals.

Now maximize what you have learned so that you can develop the muscle mass and strength that you want to achieve all while avoiding injuries.

Keep in mind to reference the pictures in this book for each workout so that you are able to visually see how each workout should be properly done.

Also, keep in mind the number of repetitions you would like to perform in order to achieve your strength training goals.

Remember 1 to 5 repetitions builds pure raw strength while 6-12 repetitions build muscle, strength and endurance.

In addition, 12 or more repetitions build muscular endurance and size.

I wish you great success with achieving your health and fitness goals.

Make sure to read the **"Health and Fitness Chief Aim"** on the following page.

Health and Fitness
Chief Aim

*Use the following guide for achieving your health and fitness goals.

Step #1
Write down your health and fitness goal(s) and be specific. For example, if you want to lose 10 pounds then write down, "I want to lose 10 pounds."

At the same time, if you want to build muscle, be specific and write down the amount of muscle you want to have. For example, if you want to have 10 pounds of muscle then write down, "I want to have 10 pounds of muscle."

Step #2
Write down the date by which you want to achieve your health and fitness goal(s).

For example, "I will lose 10 pounds by February 2019."

Example two, "I will be able to run 15 miles nonstop by May 2019."

Step 3
Write down what you are willing to sacrifice in order to achieve your health and fitness goals. In addition, write down what are you willing to give back (to the world) in return for achieving your health and fitness goal(s).

For example, "I am willing to give up drinking alcohol, specifically beer for the next 3 months in order to lose 20 pounds of fat. In addition,

I am going to stop watching television after 10:00 PM and I will instead go to sleep early so that I can wake up early and exercise."

"In return for achieving my health and fitness goals, I will serve as a role model inspiring and helping others to also achieve their health and fitness goals by sharing my knowledge, experience and wisdom."

Step 4

Repeat looking and reading over your Health and Fitness Chief Aim every day until you achieve your health and fitness goals. In addition, look and read over your Health and Fitness Chief Aim multiple times a day. Daily repetition is important for achieving any goal.

Made in the USA
Columbia, SC
02 June 2019